Pediatric Audiology

Current Trends

Editor in chief, Speech, Language, and Hearing Disorders Series
William H. Perkins, PhD

Pediatric Audiology

Current Trends

edited by

James Jerger, PhD
**Department of Otorhinolaryngology &
Communicative Sciences
Baylor College of Medicine**

COLLEGE-HILL PRESS, San Diego, California

College-Hill Press
4284 41st Street
San Diego, California 92105

Library of Congress Cataloging in Publication Data

Main entry under title:
Pediatric audiology.

  Bibliography: p.
  Includes index.
  1. Hearing disorders in children — Diagnosis.
2. Audiometry. 3. Audiology. I. Jerger, James.
[DNLM: 1. Audiometry — In infancy and childhood.
2. Child health services — In infancy and childhood.
3. Hearing disorders — In infancy and childhood.
4. Hearing disorders — Rehabilitation. WV 271 P3714]
RF291.5.C45P433 1983   618.92'0978   83–7659
ISBN 0-933014-99-6

Printed in the United States of America

Publisher's Note

These volumes were developed under the supervision of a group of leading scientists charged with the responsibility of assessing the most critical book needs of the speech-language-hearing profession. In consultation with William H. Perkins and Raymond G. Daniloff, serving as editors in chief of the ensuing volumes on speech, language, and hearing disorders (Perkins) and speech, language, and hearing science (Daniloff), the publisher planned a series of nine mutually independent texts covering the entirety of state-of-the-art knowledge in these disciplines, with contributions by respected, productive, and current scholars known for their expertise as specialists in key areas.

Each contribution has been stringently refereed for content, pedagogy, and practical value for students and practitioners by the individual volume editors, Charles Berlin, Janis Costello, Raymond Daniloff, Audrey Holland, James Jerger, Rita Naremore, and their designated reviewers, in close consultation throughout with the editors in chief and the publisher. Users are thus assured that their needs for accurate, timely information, reflecting the highest standards of scholarship and professionalism, have been faithfully met.

On behalf of the speech-language-hearing profession, its researchers, teachers, practitioners, and students, present and future, the publisher thanks the more than 100 authors and editors who have given generously of their time and knowledge to produce this magnificent contribution to the literature.

Pediatric Audiology, edited by James Jerger, is one of nine state-of-the-art volumes comprising the College-Hill Press series covering the current body of knowledge in speech, language, and hearing.

Volume Titles:	Editors:
Speech Disorders in Children	Janis Costello
Speech Disorders in Adults	Janis Costello
Speech Science	Raymond Daniloff
Language Disorders in Children	Audrey Holland
Language Disorders in Adults	Audrey Holland
Language Science	Rita Naremore
Pediatric Audiology	James Jerger
Hearing Disorders in Adults	James Jerger
Hearing Science	Charles Berlin

Editor in chief, Speech, Language, and Hearing Disorders Series: William H. Perkins

Editor in chief, Speech, Language, and Hearing Science Series: Raymond G. Daniloff

Contents

Contributors

Fred H. Bess, PhD
Vanderbilt University School of
Medicine
Bill Wilkerson Hearing & Speech
Center
Nashville, TN 37232

Rebecca M. Fischer
Vanderbilt University School of
Medicine
Bill Wilkerson Hearing & Speech
Center
Nashville, TN 37232

Susan Jerger, MS
Department of
Otorhinolaryngology &
Communicative Sciences
Baylor College of Medicine
Houston, TX 77030

Susan A. Logan, MS
Vanderbilt University School of
Medicine
Bill Wilkerson Hearing & Speech
Center
Nashville, TN 37232

Karla S. MacKimmie, MA
The Shea Clinic & Deafness
Foundation
Memphis, TN 38104

Noel D. Matkin, PhD
Department of Speech & Hearing
Sciences
University of Arizona
Tucson, AZ 85721

Freeman McConnell, PhD
Vanderbilt University School of
Medicine
The Bill Wilkerson Hearing &
Speech Center
Nashville, TN 37232

Daniel J. Orchik, PhD
The Shea Clinic & Deafness
Foundation
Memphis, TN 38104

Jon F. Peters, PhD
Nicolet Biomedical
5225 Verona Road
Madison, WI 53711

Gary Thompson, PhD
Department of Speech &
Hearing Sciences
University of Washington
Seattle, WA 98195

Wesley R. Wilson, PhD
Department of Speech &
Hearing Sciences
University of Washington
Seattle, WA 98195

Don W. Worthington, PhD
Boys Town Institute for
Communication Disorders in
Children
Omaha, NB 68131

Foreword

From 1977 to 1982, while editing the *Journal of Speech and Hearing Disorders,* I became increasingly aware of the rate at which information about communication disorders was expanding. Not only was it an information explosion, it was a conceptual explosion as well, particularly in the area of children's language. We are departing rapidly from a relatively insular profession in which clinical practice has been based largely on what we could learn from our own experience. What we are moving toward is a theory-based profession in which we are open to broad-ranging conceptions, most notably from linguistics, medicine, and psychology.

It was against this background that *Recent Advances: Speech, Language, and Hearing Disorders* was spawned. In accepting the responsibility of being editor in chief, I saw several opportunities. Above all, it offered a vehicle by which the profession could remain current. Some areas have moved so rapidly that they bear little resemblance to what they were even a decade ago. Not only has information proliferated, but so have the journals and texts in which it has been preserved. Here, then, in *Recent Advances,* was an opportunity to organize a coherent and comprehensive account of the current state of affairs in all clinical aspects of speech, language, and hearing.

A price paid for advancement of knowledge is not only inability to consume the increasing glut, but even to comprehend it. One must almost be a specialist to understand what other specialists are talking about. To chronicle the state of the art across all areas of communication disorders, and still make responsible statements, would require the best minds available in each area. To know who the experts in these areas are, and to obtain their participation, would require scholars of such stature as to attract them. Hence, my most important responsibility in this project was the selection of volume editors. I take great pride that Janis Costello, Audrey Holland, and James Jerger agreed to participate.

With their respective editorships established, my remaining responsibility was to consult with them in determining the chapters needed to report the state of the art in their areas, and in selecting authors most qualified to prepare the chapters. We sought authors who not only are established scholars, but who also write with clarity. We were as concerned that anyone in the profession be able to read and understand what is going on in any area as we were with assembling the best information available. Aside from nudging the project along occasionally and final editing, I can claim little credit for the sterling quality of these texts. That credit belongs to the editors.

William H. Perkins
Editor in chief

Preface

The past decade has seen revolutionary changes in pediatric evaluation. Two new techniques, immittance audiometry and auditory brain stem response, have freed us from our previously total dependence on behavioral audiometry. The result has been two-fold; first, a gradual decrease in the minimum age at which the hearing of children can be tested and, second, a gradual increase in the accuracy of our diagnostic evaluations.

During this same period, we have seen major legislative changes affecting all handicapped children. Public Law 94-142 has had a broad impact on habilitation services for all hearing-impaired children.

This book was conceived in an attempt to summarize these major new developments and to place them in the perspective of clinical practice. We review contemporary trends under three subheadings: diagnostic evaluation, amplification, and habilitation. Within each subheading, we have attempted to focus on contemporary trends and newer concepts rather than on an exhaustive review of the state of the art. And, indeed, it should become apparent that concepts and techniques unique to only the past decade dominate the state of the art in many areas.

It is difficult to judge which of the many advances in pediatric evaluation and management has had greatest impact during the past decade. My own vote goes to immittance audiometry. As Orchik and MacKimmie so well summarize in their chapter, immittance measures now pervade pediatric testing. The combination of tympanogram and acoustic reflex provides an unrivaled tool for detecting and monitoring middle ear disease, the scourge of hearing in childhood. With techniques unavailable less than 20 years ago, we can screen for middle ear disorder in a pediatric population as young as 3–6 months, we can monitor progress in treatment, and we can maintain virtually constant surveillance of severely impaired children where the additional 10–20 dB in lost sensitivity imposed by a transient episode of otitis media may have extremely serious consequences both in the classroom and in daily social intercourse.

For the clinician, immittance audiometry has provided a powerful cross-check on other measures of auditory sensitivity in young children. In combination with ABR, it has brought considerable improvement to the accuracy and efficiency of pediatric audiologic evaluation.

But, perhaps the most significant contribution of immittance audiometry has been its role in emphasizing the hitherto neglected consequence of mild fluctuating sensitivity loss on the acquisition of speech and language skills in young children. By focusing attention on the child with recurrent bouts of otitis media, on the prevalence of the disorder, and on the nature and degree of the auditory sequelae, immittance audiometry has stimulated a broad spectrum of research, much of it still controversial, but interwoven with an inevitable conclusion that, during the critical language-learning period, even mild transient sensitivity loss can have deleterious effects far beyond our most pessimistic expectations two decades ago.

If immittance audiometry has had the greatest impact on the pediatric population, the auditory brain stem response is certainly a close second. Worthington and Peters, at Boys Town, have been in a position uniquely suited to evaluate the impact on this new tool in the testing of children. They discuss a broad spectrum of applications, from the neonatal intensive care unit to the child with speech and/or language delay. While there can be no doubt that ABR has virtually revolutionized pediatric testing, Worthington and Peters quite correctly remind us that the interpretation of ABR, and indeed all evoked potential data, can be misleading when analyzed in isolation, and is best viewed in relation to the total audiologic and neurologic evaluation of the child.

In spite of the impressive advances provided by electroacoustic and electrophysiologic techniques, it is well to remind ourselves that behavioral audiometry is, and will probably always be, the method of choice for evaluating total auditory function. Wilson and Thompson catalogue impressive advances in behavior measures of auditory sensitivity. They summarize exciting evidence that visual reinforcement techniques can be successfully applied to children as young as 6 months.

In a similar vein, Susan Jerger shows how quite sophisticated suprathreshold measures of speech understanding can be successfully applied to children as young as 36 months. These impressive advances in both threshold and suprathreshold audiometry have the potential to increase the scope of behavioral evaluation to include not only measures of peripheral sensitivity, but measures of central auditory processing as well.

The key to the successful exploitation of all these advances in our routine clinical work lies, perhaps, in the development of newer strategies for using them in judicious combination. We may anticipate, for example, that refined behavioral measures of auditory sensitivity, combined with the cross-check capability and precision of immittance audiometry, and the stability and precision of ABR, will ultimately provide a quantum leap over the strategies of only a decade ago in the accuracy and reliability with which peripheral hearing loss can be predicted.

Similarly, the combination of advanced speech audiometry and the total auditory-evoked potential examination, including ABR, middle, and late potentials, will ultimately lead to much better understanding of central auditory disorders, their relation to language and learning disorders, their prevalence in children with impaired peripheral function, and their impact on the habilitation of the hearing-impaired child.

The past decade has seen several important advances in our approach to the management and habilitation of hearing-impaired children. Matkin's summary of changes in our thinking about hearing aids for children, for example, emphasizes the importance of amplification for mild loss to a degree not sufficiently appreciated even 10 years ago.

Bess and Logan review the many issues relating to auditory trainers and other educational amplification devices. Their chapter includes a discussion of infrared transmission systems, a technology which is certain to have a profound effect on classrooms and other amplification environments.

In the habilitation area, Fischer reviews the persistent unresolved issues in the educational programming of hearing-impaired children and emphasizes the importance of assessment in designing programs best suited to optimizing the learning environment of the individual child.

Finally, McConnell reviews the events leading up to the legislative landmark, PL #94-142, and its impact on the provision of services to the hearing-handicapped child.

My own reading of these interesting chapters leaves me with two strong impressions. First, we are doing an incredibly better job on children than many thought possible as recently as 10 years ago. We can now test children's hearing at virtually any age, and we are even beginning to separate peripheral from central components.

Equally strong, however, is the impression that we have only begun to exploit the new techniques now available to us. In many areas of habilitation, for example, recent advances in both electrophysiologic and behavioral testing have not yet been successfully applied. There remains an urgent need to translate the findings from research laboratories, and the experiences of large clinical centers, to the less dramatic but overridingly important historic problems faced by all those who work with the day-to-day problems of hearing-impaired children.

James Jerger
Editor

Wesley R. Wilson
Gary Thompson

Behavioral Audiometry

Introduction

Recent advances in behavioral audiometry for children have centered on improved assessment procedures for infants. This focus has not been accidental. Hearing loss, depending on severity, age of onset, and a host of other factors, has a mild-to-profound impact on communicative functioning. Accordingly, it is crucial that hearing impairment be identified, defined, and managed prior to the language-learning period in order to foster optimal growth in communication skills. Prior to about 1970, it generally was believed that only gross behavioral hearing tests could be obtained on infants 2 years of age and younger. Refinements in methodology have occurred over the past few years which have dramatically altered this view, as well as allowing us to better understand the auditory abilities of infants. It is now becoming possible to obtain rather complete behavioral assessment of auditory function in infants 6 months through 2 years of age.

Behavioral assessment of auditory thresholds of infants is based on observation of overt responses to controlled auditory signals. There are two general approaches which have been used clinically. They can be differentiated by whether or not reinforcement is employed. When no reinforcement is used, the procedure is usually called behavior observation audiometry (BOA). As the name implies, this is a passive approach. The examiner observes changes in behavior (responses) which are time-locked to auditory signals, but does not assume an active "teaching" role. As an estimator of hearing sensitivity, the BOA procedure has inherent limitations because infant responses are not brought under stimulus control by the examiner. For neonates, suprathreshold stimulation is required to elicit reflexive responses such as startle or eye widening. Older infants demonstrate "awareness" or spontaneous head-turn responses at reasonably low intensity levels (Downs & Sterritt, 1967; Suzuki & Sato, 1961; Thompson & Thompson, 1972), but the probability of obtaining a response is dependent on the nature of the auditory stimulus (Eisenberg, 1976; Hoversten & Moncur, 1969; Ling, Ling, & Doehring, 1970; Thompson & Thompson, 1972), response habituation is likely (Moore, Thompson, & Thompson, 1975), and variability is high (Thompson & Weber, 1974). Even though BOA lacks precision as an indicator of hearing status, it is the only available behavioral procedure for some profoundly retarded children, or very young infants who cannot be conditioned to respond to auditory signals.

When reinforcement is employed, the testing approach is a form of operant conditioning in which the auditory signal (discriminative stimulus) cues the availability of reinforcement following the desired response behavior. The age at which infants can be conditioned to respond to auditory signals is of continuing interest to many investigators. Over the past decade or so, the literature in the area of speech perception has provided support for the notion that infants possess far more sophisticated auditory abilities than previously had been suspected (Eilers, 1978; Kuhl, 1980; Morse, 1978). Central to this theme is the thesis that the infant is an active receptor of auditory information, who, if given the chance, will interact with, and control, his or her auditory environment. Behavioral test procedures that acknowledge and capitalize on this fact provide more powerful indices of auditory function in infants than behavioral procedures that view the infant as a passive reactor to sound.

Among conditioning procedures for infants, visual reinforcement audiometry (VRA) has emerged as a successful assessment tool for infants 6 months through 2 years of age. In this procedure, head turns toward a sound source are reinforced by an attractive visual stimulus (animated toy). The success of this procedure, no doubt, is related to the fact that the response (head turn) and reinforcer (animated toy) are geared well to the developmental level of young infants. At 6 months of age, virtually all normally developing infants have learned to turn in the direction of "interesting" sounds in their environment. Thus, in the testing situation, the head-turn response can often be elicited spontaneously to the initial auditory presentation, and need only be maintained through reinforcement.

Concerning reinforcement, even casual observation of infant behavior leads to the conclusion that visual stimuli are of "interest" to this age group. Babies attend to visual stimuli and generally are entertained by the myriad of toys presented to them in their natural environments. It is not surprising, then, that visual stimuli serve a reinforcing function for auditory responses obtained in a formal hearing-test situation.

This chapter has three purposes. The first is to summarize the results of studies of infant audition that have used BOA or nonreinforced behavioral procedures. Since this literature serves as the base for much of the current thinking concerning infant auditory abilities, it is important to understand some of the potential shortcomings in the procedure. The second purpose of the chapter is to detail the research literature that forms the basis for behavioral procedures employing reinforcement with particular emphasis on VRA. The third purpose is to discuss the application of VRA to clinical cases.

Behavior Observation Audiometry

Neonates

The use of behavior observation audiometry (BOA) with neonates and very young infants requires attention to a number of factors. Eisenberg (1976) has provided an excellent review. First, the state of the infant has a major effect on responsiveness. For example, in rating sleep in stages from deep sleep to fully awake, it has been demonstrated that the middle states allow the highest response ratios. In terms of signal factors, Eisenberg (1976) reports that band-pass signals are better than pure tones; that low-frequency signals soothe the infant, whereas high-frequency signals distress the infant; that the response ratio of the infant increases with signal duration; and that rapid rise-time signals produce defense reflexes, whereas slow rise-time signals produce orienting responses. The factors used in determining a response are generally reflexive behaviors—for example, eye widening, blink, and arousal. Because a wide variety of response behaviors is monitored, one major difficulty is the fact that the tester may be influenced by preinformation bias—that is, the examiner's expectations of the outcome of the test. For example, if an infant is seen for whom the history includes a normal APGAR, and normal pregnancy and family history, the expectation of the examiner is somewhat different than in the case of an infant born to deaf parents. Likewise, another form of bias may occur in the test situation. When the examiner is aware of the sound stimuli presentations, he or she adopts a different criterion in defining infant responses than in test protocols where the examiner does not know when sound is presented, and "blind" control (no-sound) intervals are included. Moncur (1968), Weber (1969, 1970), and Goldstein and Tait (1971) have each discussed the potential effects of these forms of preinformation bias; Weber (1969) and Goldstein and Tait (1971) suggest procedural approaches that may reduce or remove the effects of these several types of bias. One difficulty that remains, however, is the fact that the signal levels used in BOA testing with neonates would, at best, identify only those infants with severe-to-profound losses. The testing does not provide results that allow adequate description of an infant's auditory function, nor any substantial information concerning habilitative needs.

Infants and Young Children

Beyond the newborn period, a number of sources have described the application of BOA procedures to the developing infant. The procedures generally are discussed in terms of effectiveness of different signal types, the "development" of responses in infants, and the signal levels necessary to produce a response. A major emphasis is often placed on the " development" of the auditory response as a function of the signal level necessary to elicit a response. An example of this approach is illustrated in Northern and Downs (1978). They report that between the newborn period and 4 months of age, the normal infant is aroused from sleep by sound signals of 90 dB SPL in a noisy environment and 50–70 dB SPL in a quiet environment. They indicate that at approximately 3 to 4 months of age the normal infant begins to make a rudimentary head turn toward a sound signal of 50–60 dB SPL. From 4 to 7 months, the infant turns directly to the side of signal presentation at a level of 40–50 dB SPL. From 7 to 9 months, the infant directly locates a sound source of 30–40 dB to the side and below. From 9 to 13 months, the infant locates a sound source of 25–35 dB SPL to the side and below. From 13 to 16 months, the infant localizes sound signals of 25–30 dB SPL to the side, below, and indirectly above. And from 16 months to 21 months, the vertical localization improves. As can be seen in this sequence, reported by Northern and Downs (1978), the infant is depicted as showing a development of the localization response, as well as a marked shift in the level of signal necessary to produce the response. This has led many practitioners to talk in terms of a rather pronounced development of auditory sensitivity in the first few years of life.

Another example of similar information is provided by Sweitzer (1977), and is shown in Figure 1-1. The minimal response level for speech is depicted as shifting from 70 dB SPL for a neonate, to 45 dB SPL for a 6-month-old infant, and finally reaching a response level similar to adults at 24

FIGURE 1-1
Response Levels for Speech as a Function of Age (From R.S. Sweitzer, in *Hearing Loss in Children* edited by B.F. Jaffe, 1977.)

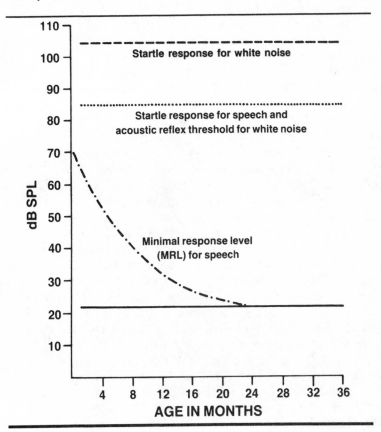

months of age. Put another way, the minimal response level for speech is shown to shift approximately 45 to 50 dB during the first two years of life. Again, this finding has sometimes been overinterpreted to mean that the infant's hearing sensitivity is shifting by this amount during the two years of infancy.

With reference to the issue of development of localization, Muir and Field and colleagues (Field, Difranco, Dodwell, & Muir, 1979; Field, Muir, Pilon, Sinclair, & Dodwell, 1980; Muir, Abraham, Forbes, & Harris, 1979; Muir & Field, 1979) have presented an interesting series of studies demonstrating that neonates consistently will turn their heads toward a sound source. Their experimental procedure involved the use of video scoring and other controls for potential observer bias. In most cases, the latency of the neonates' responses was long—2.5 secs to the beginning of the head-turn response and 5.5 secs to the end of the response. Another finding of interest in their longitudinal study of infants was that the localization responses tended to decline at 2-3 months of age and return strongly at 4 months. Comparing these collective findings of Muir and colleagues to the literature in pediatric audiology, one is struck by the fact that our ideas about the development of localization responses may have seriously underestimated the actual abilities of infants. To our knowledge, no clinical application of the work of Muir et al. has been undertaken yet, and it is to be emphasized that their studies were for the purpose of studying the localization behavior of infants. The findings remain provocative, however.

Another major theme in the BOA literature is the relative effectiveness of different signals, again as a function of age. Figure 1-2, from Northern and Downs (1978), provides one summary of this type of information. Observe, for example, the 4-7 month age frame, and note that an infant will respond to speech at 21 dB relative to normal adult thresholds, while responding to warbled pure tones at 51 dB relative to audiometric zero. This difference of 30 dB is an indication of the relative inefficiency of warbled pure tones for producing appropriate auditory thresholds using a BOA approach. Figure 1-2 illustrates again the rather marked changes in signal intensities necessary to produce responses over the first two years of life with the BOA procedure. Using warbled pure tones as an example, the shift is 52 dB. This shift has been discussed from the point of view of "auditory development." We will attempt, in this chapter, to develop an interpretation that depicts the major portion of this shift as being a function of test methodology, and not of marked changes in true hearing sensitivity.

In another study on the relative effectiveness of different test stimuli with infants, Thompson and Thompson (1972) compared a speech signal, filtered speech signal, white noise, filtered white noise, and a 3000 Hz pure tone. As is evident in Figure 1-3, the speech signal produced the highest percentage of responses in infants 7–12 months of age, with the pure tone producing the fewest responses. For the most part, the signals showed similar efficiency regardless of the presentation level of the signal. Note, however, that in this BOA procedure the most efficient signal, speech, produced fewer than 50% responses at an HL of 15 dB in infants aged 7–12 months. Looking at results from the same study with older infants in Figure 1-4, one again finds a clear difference in the effectiveness of various signals, with speech producing the highest percentage of responses and the 3000 Hz pure tone producing the fewest responses. For the older infants, the overall percentage of response is increased for all signals as compared to

FIGURE 1-2
Response Levels as a Function of Signal and Age (From J. L. Northern and M. P. Downs, 1978.)

Age	Noisemakers (Approx. SPL)	Warbled Pure Tones (Re: Audiometric Zero)	Speech (Re: Audiometric Zero)
0 wk. - 6 wk.	50-70 dB	78 dB (SD = 6 dB)	40-60 dB
6 wk. - 4 mo.	50-60 dB	70 dB (SD = 10 dB)	47 dB (SD = 2 dB)
4 mo. - 7 mo.	40-50 dB	51 dB (SD = 9 dB)	21 dB (SD = 8 dB)
7 mo. - 9 mo.	30-40 dB	45 dB (SD = 15 dB)	15 dB (SD = 7 dB)
9 mo. - 13 mo.	25-35 dB	38 dB (SD = 8 dB)	8 dB (SD = 7 dB)
13 mo. - 16 mo.	25-30 dB	32 dB (SD = 10 dB)	5 dB (SD = 5 dB)
16 mo. - 21 mo.	25 dB	25 dB (SD = 10 dB)	5 dB (SD = 1 dB)
21 mo. - 24 mo.	25 dB	26 dB (SD = 10 dB)	3 dB (SD = 2 dB)

the younger infants. Note, however, that for even the most efficient signals, the response rate remains at a level of 65–75% for signals at 15 dB HL in this unreinforced test paradigm.

Another area of concern involving the BOA procedure is that of intra- and intersubject variability. Thompson and Weber (1974) presented data on both topics. Using a band-pass filtered complex-noise signal, they reported intrasubject variability of more than 20 dB for three signal presentations in one-third of their subjects, ranging in age from 3 months through 5 years. Generally, Trial 1 produced the best threshold, with succeedingly poorer (higher) thresholds in Trials 2 and 3. The clinical import of this finding is that use of the BOA procedure allows one a very limited number of responses for answering clinical questions. Furthermore, the wide intrasubject variability makes it difficult to consider test-retest situations—for example, in monitoring the effectiveness of drug therapy in treatment of middle ear problems.

FIGURE 1-3
Percentage Response to Five Stimuli as a Function of Hearing Level—7 to 12 Months of Age (From M. Thompson and G. Thompson, 1972.)

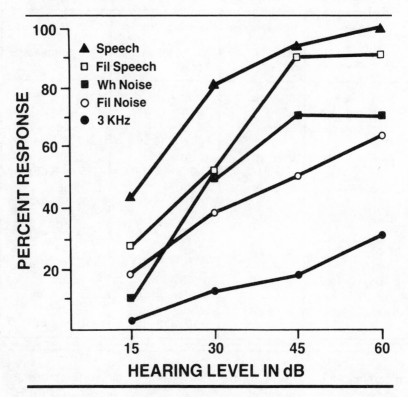

In terms of intersubject variability, the same study (Thompson & Weber, 1974) illustrated a wide spread in obtained BOA "thresholds" from presumed normal-hearing infants and young children of similar ages. For example, in the age bracket of 3 to 5 months, the dispersion between the 10th and 90th percentile is on the order of 65 dB, as can be seen in Figure 1-5. In the age category from 6 through 18 months, the dispersion remains substantial. This wide intersubject variability is one of the major limiting factors in the use of BOA. If a population of normally developing infants yields a range of responses that encompasses nearly the total measurement range used in hearing assessment, it is impossible to define hearing loss as a change or deviation from this "norm." Put another way, the essence of hearing assessment is to find a procedure and signal that yield a very tight grouping of scores for a normal population, with a wide range

FIGURE 1-4
Percentage Response to Five Stimuli as a Function of Hearing Level—22 to 36 Months of Age (From M. Thompson and G. Thompson, 1972.)

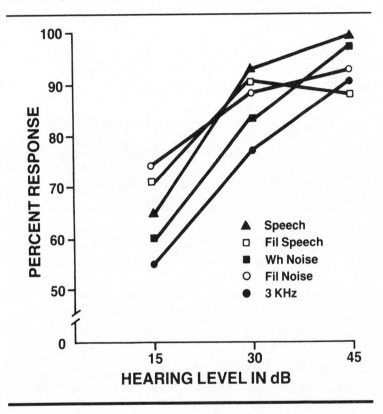

available for defining abnormal scores. The BOA procedure does not meet this goal. As Thompson and Weber point out in their study:

BOA thresholds may well tend to underestimate the extent of a child's hearing. That is, the child who does not respond below 50 dB HL may well have a "true threshold" somewhat below this level. Unfortunately, there is no way to determine an appropriate correction factor for an individual child. Put in proper perspective, BOA is probably best viewed as a screening assessment procedure (p. 2).

Finally, the problem of observer bias again manifests itself with clinical populations of older children. Gans and Flexer (1982) studied observer bias in the BOA testing of profoundly involved multiply handicapped children and reported clear bias effects in the testing of 85% of the children as a

FIGURE 1-5
Intersubject Variability in BOA as a Function of Age (From G. Thompson and B. A. Weber, 1974.)

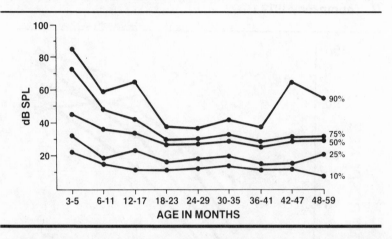

function of the examiners being aware of the stimulus type and intensity. They suggest that the effects of this particular form of bias can be reduced by using a video-scoring procedure in which the examiners are denied knowledge of stimulus events.

Interpretations of previous behavioral data, generated through use of the BOA procedure, result in the following summary statements:

1. The potential for observer bias in judging responses complicates the task;
2. The obtained thresholds improve substantially as a function of age;
3. The obtained thresholds vary substantially as a function of signal used—pure tones are not an effective signal;
4. Infants and young children habituate to the test stimulus, which results in large intrasubject variability in a substantial number of cases; and
5. A substantial variability in threshold estimates occurs across infants—this variability makes it difficult to establish "norms" using the BOA procedure.

Operant Conditioning

Among the difficulties that occur as a result of use of BOA, two factors stand out. The first is that a variety of responses is used, making response judgment problematic. The second is that any pediatric audiometric test procedure is dependent upon the infant continuing to show consistent responses to sound over a number of presentations. In the BOA procedure, it is apparent that sound is not a highly motivating signal for continued or consistent response behavior. First, the infant does not necessarily respond at or near threshold and, second, the infant quickly habituates to repeated signal presentations.

In order to overcome these shortcomings, it is possible to consider the selection of a single response coupled with reinforcement to increase the number of responses. Two operant conditioning approaches have been used for this purpose—conjugate procedures and operant discrimination procedures. In conjugate procedures, the stimulus follows the response as a consequence and is the reinforcer. Conversely, in an operant discrimination paradigm, the stimulus is used to cue the infant that a response will produce reinforcement. Any reinforcer may be used.

Conjugate Procedures

An example of application of the conjugate procedure is contained in a study by Eisele, Berry, and Shriner (1975). They connected a nonnutritive nipple (pacifier), used as a pressure transducer, to a Bekesy-type audiometer so that the sucking behavior of the infant would control the intensity of the pulsed pure-tone signals. The signal was delivered through a loudspeaker positioned over the infant's crib. This conjugate procedure allowed the intensity of a continuously available reinforcing stimulus to vary as a function of the sucking-response rate. Sucking rates equal to or higher than baseline rates resulted in a 5 dB/sec intensity increase; cessation of sucking resulted in an intensity decrease. Figure 1-6 shows a tracing from a 36-hour-old infant (from Eisele, Berry, and Shriner, 1975) which demonstrates five reversals or cessations of sucking; the arrows correspond to behavioral responses scored by observers as a means of a validity judgment. Certain infants were also seen 24 hours later and produced comparable results. It is interesting to note that although this procedure was described in 1975, the results have not been replicated to our knowledge, and it has not been adapted as a procedure for clinical evaluation of neonates. Friedlander (1969, 1970) also has described the application of conjugate procedures in what he calls "the playtest for selective listening."

A major drawback of conjugate procedures for threshold determination is the fact that the sound stimuli used for assessment are not particularly reinforcing for normally developing infants. Since conjugate procedures require that the stimulus serve as a reinforcer, this may be considered a fatal drawback in terms of their usefulness as a clinical test of

FIGURE 1-6
Bekesy Tracings From Sucking Behavior of a 36-hour-old Infant
(From W. A. Eisele, R. C. Berry, and T. H. Shriner, 1975.)

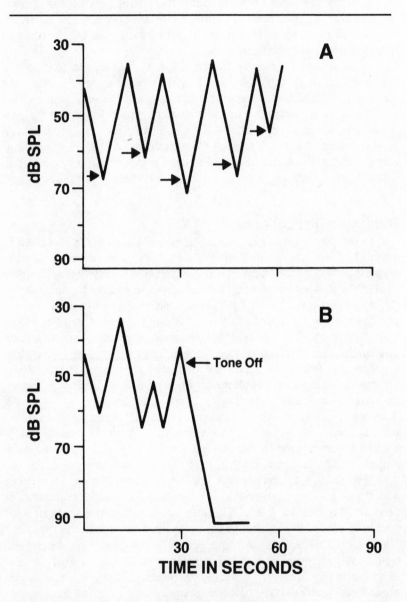

Note: Arrows indicate behavioral responses.

auditory threshold. However, the conjugate procedures might have considerable application to tasks of auditory preference accomplished at suprathreshold levels.

Operant Discrimination Procedures

As noted above, in this category of procedures the stimulus is independent of the reinforcer—the stimulus cues the infant that a response will immediately produce reinforcement. One is free to select the most potent reinforcer for the particular age category being tested. Throughout the remainder of this chapter we will describe a number of applications of the operant discrimination paradigm. Considering the operant discrimination procedure from the point of view of responses and reinforcers, we have made use of the following:

> *Responses (operants)*
> 1. Leg swing
> 2. Head turn
> 3. Bar press
>
> *Reinforcers*
> 1. None
> 2. Social
> 3. Visual-social
> 4. Edible-social

In selecting a response to use with the procedure, one obviously must consider the neuromuscular development of the infant to be tested. Among the response repertoire available, the leg swing can be used with very young infants; a head turn is a natural response mode for infants aged 4 to 6 months and older (see, however, our previous comments on "auditory localization"); and the bar-press response has been used with infants as young as 7–8 months and older. The leg-swing response has not been used extensively, nor does it, at present, seem applicable in the clinical process because a substantial number of training sessions are required to bring the response under stimulus control.

The head-turn response has been used extensively. Figures 1-7A through 1-7C illustrate a common use of this in the visually reinforced audiometry (VRA) task. In Figure 1-7A, the assistant holds the infant's attention at midline. When the infant is in a response-ready state, a sound is introduced, in this case through a loudspeaker to the left of the infant at an angle

14   Wilson/Thompson

FIGURE 1-7A
VRA procedure-assistant maintains the infant's attention at midline.

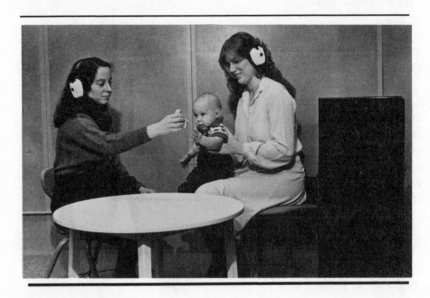

FIGURE 1-7B
VRA procedure - head-turn response.

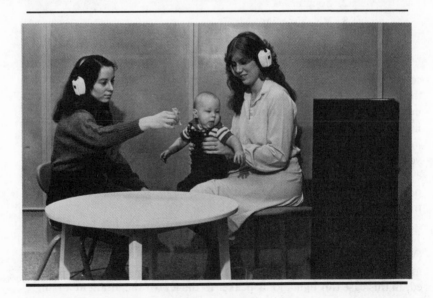

FIGURE 1-7C
VRA procedure - visual reinforcement.

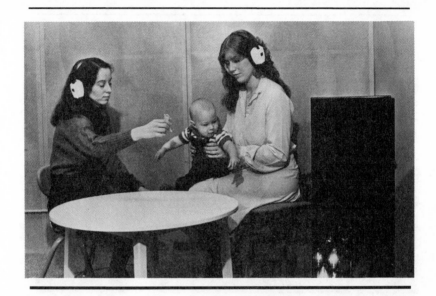

of approximately 45° from the midline position. Figure 1-7B shows the head-turn response followed by the visual reinforcer in Figure 1-7C.

Use of the bar-press procedure, coupled with food reinforcement, sometimes called TROCA (Tangible Reinforcement Operant Conditioning Audiometry) is illustrated in Figures 1-8A through 1-8D. In Figure 1-8A, the sound stimulus has been presented, and the infant responds by pressing the manipulandum. The correct response coupled to the stimulus presentation results in reinforcement—Figure 1-8B. The reinforcement includes a light to draw the infant's attention to the area where the food is presented, and then the food bit. Figures 1-8C and 1-8D show completion of the process. In Figure 1-9, the bar-press response is shown as coupled with a visual reinforcer sometimes called VROCA (Visual Reinforcement Operant Conditioning Audiometry). In this case, a correct response (hit) provides a short duration of visual reinforcement.

Visual Reinforcement Audiometry

Historical Perspective

Normally developing infants make head turns toward a sound source in the first few months of life. The localization response represents a

FIGURE 1-8A
TROCA procedure - infant presses manipulandum.

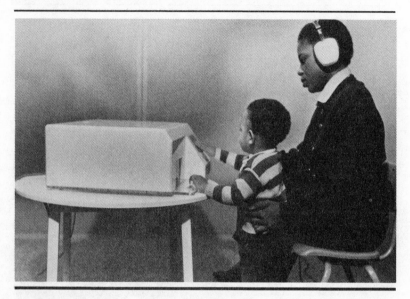

FIGURE 1-8B
TROCA procedure - food reinforcement.

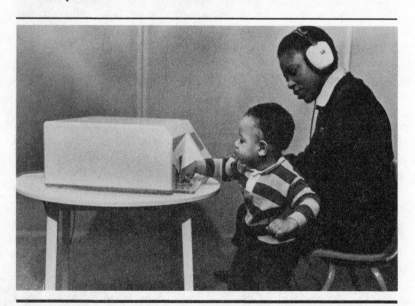

FIGURE 1-8C
TROCA procedure - infant completes task.

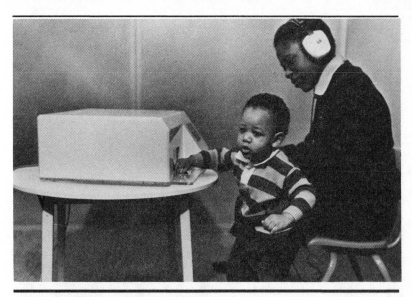

FIGURE 1-8D
TROCA procedure - infant completes task.

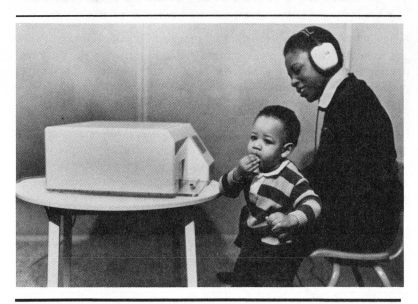

FIGURE 1-9
VROCA procedure - bar-press response with visual reinforcement.

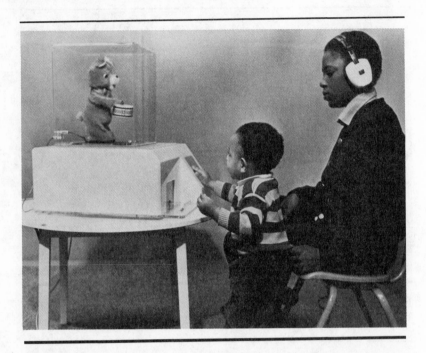

behavioral "window" through which many aspects of auditory behavior can be studied. If an infant's localization behavior deviates markedly from the normal developmental pattern, there is strong reason to suspect the presence of either hearing loss or other problems, such as mental retardation. While there is a decided tendency for infants to turn initially toward "interesting" or "novel" auditory stimuli, there is a limit to the number of times head turns will occur to repeated stimuli (Moore, Thompson, & Thompson, 1975; Moore, Wilson, & Thompson, 1977). From a hearing-assessment standpoint, habituation of response to repeated stimulus presentations is undesirable because it reduces the number of stimulus trials available for threshold determination.

Suzuki and Ogiba (1960, 1961) were the first to report on a conditioning procedure involving the localization response. The procedure was called *conditioned orientation reflex* (COR) audiometry and was based on the observation that infants will reflexively turn their heads toward a strange auditory or visual stimulus. In the initial stages of conditioning, a pure tone was presented through a loudspeaker at an intensity level estimated to be 30 to 40 dB above the infant's threshold. One second later a visual stimulus (illuminated doll) was presented from the same location. The combined tone and light stimulus lasted for about 4 seconds. After a few conditioning trials, the timing sequence was changed so that the visual stimulus followed the auditory stimulus and was presented only if the child had first responded to the tone. It was presumed that the visual stimulus served to reinforce head-turn responses leading to successful threshold estimates for over 80% of children in the 1- to 3-year age category. The success rate was less than 50% for infants under 1 year of age.

Liden and Kankkunen (1969) were the first to use the term *visual reinforcement audiometry* (VRA) to describe a modified COR procedure which they developed. Since they accepted any type of response behavior that could be judged (at least for young infants), and always provided "reinforcement," their procedure differed markedly from that described by Suzuki and Ogiba. Even though Liden and Kankkunen used the term VRA to describe a specific test protocol, the term has come to be used in a generic sense to describe a class of procedures involving the use of visual stimuli as reinforcers. We believe that the term VRA is more appropriate than COR for describing this general category of tests because we have been able to use the head-turn response and visual reinforcement with some infants and older retarded children who did not initially show an orienting-localization response to sound, but could be taught this response.

In addition to Suzuki and Ogiba (1960, 1961) and Liden and Kankkunen (1969), a number of authors have reported on the use of VRA procedures for assessment of hearing sensitivity in infants and young children (Haug, Baccaro, & Guilford, 1967; Motta, Facchini, & D'Auria, 1970). Generally, these studies suggest that the lower age limit for widespread use of this procedure is 12 months, although Haug, Baccaro, and Guilford (1967) reported clinical success with a small number of infants in the 5-to-12-month range.

Effectiveness of Visual Reinforcement

While the above-mentioned studies provided support for the use of VRA, there remained doubt as to the specific reinforcing value of the visual stimulus because control (no reinforcement) groups were not included for comparison results. Also, it was not clear if the type of visual stimulus employed had any bearing on its effectiveness as a reinforcer. Moore, Thompson, and Thompson (1975) studied auditory localization behavior as a function of four reinforcement conditions: (1) no reinforcement; (2) social reinforcement (a smile, verbal praise, and/or a pat on the shoulder); (3) simple visual reinforcement (a blinking red light); and (4) complex visual reinforcement (a colorful, animated toy bear that danced in place and beat a drum when activated). The subjects were 48 normal infants between 12 and 18 months of age. They were divided into groups of 12 and assigned to one of the four reinforcement conditions. Each subject sat on the parent's lap in the center of the test room. A test-room examiner kept the infant's attention focused to the front by means of soft, colorful toys. Each subject received 30 complex-noise stimulus presentations at 70 dB SPL from a loudspeaker located at a 45° angle from the infant's front line of vision. Following each appropriate head-turn response, subjects in the experimental groups received social or visual reinforcement. The control group received no reinforcement. Interspersed among the 30 test trials were 10 control trials, during which the test-room and control-room examiners recorded whether or not the infant turned toward the loudspeaker in the absence of an auditory stimulus.

Results of test trials are displayed in Figure 1-10. The mean number of responses for the complex-visual-reinforcement, simple-visual-reinforcement, social-reinforcement, and no-reinforcement groups was 27.3, 20.5, 15.2, and 9.7, respectively—all significantly different from each other. It should be noted that among the reinforcement groups, the complex reinforcement group, in particular, continued to show a high rate of response— averaging 8 responses during the last 10 stimulus presentations. In contrast, it can be seen that the control group habituated rapidly and showed only a few responses during the last 15 trials. The range of responses for the complex-reinforcement group was from 13 to 30, as contrasted to a range of 5 to 16 for the no-reinforcement group. Subjects randomly looked toward the sound source only 4.8% of the time during the control trials—that is, trials when no auditory stimulus was presented. Therefore, random behavior was ruled out as a major factor accounting for the number of positive responses obtained using the various reinforcement conditions. The results of this study indicate that auditory localization behavior of 12-to-18-month-old infants is strongly influenced by reinforcement, and that the type of reinforcement used has a systematic differentiated effect on head-turn response behavior. Visual stimuli containing movement, color, and contour are more apt to be effective reinforcers than less dimensional visual stimuli.

In a follow-up study, Moore, Wilson, and Thompson (1977) used the same complex visual reinforcer (animated toy) and a similar experimental design to explore the lower-age boundary of VRA. Sixty normal infants were divided into three groups based on age. Group 1 contained infants 7 through 11 months of age (6 months, 16 days through 11 months, 15 days), Group 2 contained 5- and 6-month olds, and Group 3 contained 4-month olds. Within each age group, there were 10 experimental subjects (visual reinforcement) and 10 control subjects (no reinforcement). Results

FIGURE 1-10
Cumulative mean head-turn responses in blocks of stimulus trials as a function of reinforcement condition - infants 12 to 18 months of age (N 5 48) (From J.M. Moore, G. Thompson, and M. Thompson, 1975.)

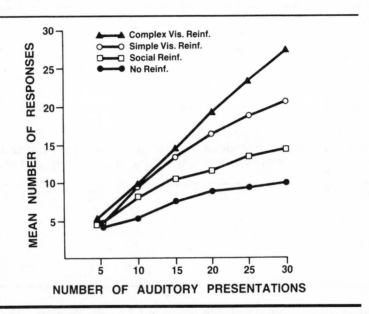

are shown in Tables 1-1 and 1-2, as well as in Figures 1-11—1-13. Differences between the experimental and control groups were significant for 7-to-11- and 5-to-6-month-old groups. The difference between groups at 4 months of age was not significant. These data imply that a complex visual stimulus can be used to reinforce localization behavior of infants as young as 5 months of age.

Whereas the previous studies explored the relative effectiveness of reinforcement and no-reinforcement conditions in a cross-sectional design, the same question can be approached in a single-subject design using a reversal paradigm. The strength of this approach rests on the fact that the subject serves as his or her own control. If reinstatement of treatment (in this case, reinforcement) following habituation of the response results in an increased rate of response, one can properly assign that effect to the treatment. Two 6-month-olds served as subjects in a study (Wilson, Moore, & Thompson, 1976) using a single-subject design. All conditions were identical to the previously described study, except for the distribution of reinforcement and no-reinforcement trials. Each subject first received 5 signal

TABLE 1-1.
Means, Standard Deviations, and Ranges of Auditory Localization Responses to 30 Signals for Experimental Groups (N = 10 in each group).

Age (months)	Mean	Standard Deviation	Range
7-11	26.6	4.1	19-30
5-6	25.5	3.8	17-30
4	6.4	12.4	0-26

TABLE 1-2.
Means, Standard Deviations, and Ranges of Auditory Localization Responses to 30 Signals for Control Groups (N = 10 in each group).

Age (months)	Mean	Standard Deviation	Range
7-11	10.7	7.9	3-25
5-6	5.5	6.5	1-19
4	7.0	8.5	0-23

presentations coupled with reinforcement for correct responses. The reinforcement contingency was then removed for the next 15 trials and, as is apparent in Figure 1-14, both infants stopped responding within that interval and their behavior stabilized in a no-response mode. On Trial 21 the visual reinforcer was coupled with the auditory signal serving as a teaching trial. For the remaining 9 trials, each correct response earned reinforcement and, as illustrated, both infants responded at a 100% rate. We feel these data provide a powerful demonstration of the strength of this reinforcement procedure for 6-month-old infants.

Soundfield Threshold Assessment

Wilson, Moore, and Thompson (1976) studied soundfield auditory thresholds using VRA. Ninety normally developing infants between 5 and 18 months were divided into groups of 15, according to age. The auditory stimulus was complex noise, and threshold sampling followed a protocol of attenuating the signal 20 dB after each positive head-turn response and increasing the signal 10 dB after each failure to respond. Control intervals

FIGURE 1-11
Cumulative mean head-turn responses in blocks of stimulus trials as a function of reinforcement condition - infants seven to 11 months of age (N = 20) (From J. M. Moore, W. R. Wilson, and G. Thompson, 1977.)

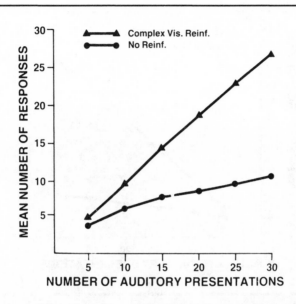

were included as before. All appropriate responses were visually reinforced (animated toy). Threshold was defined as the lowest presentation level at which the infant responded a minimum of 3 times out of a maximum of 6 signal presentations. Results are shown in Figure 1-15 and are reported in dB SPL (see endnote on page 41). As can be noted, the average response levels improved slightly with age, ranging from 21 to 29 dB SPL. The 10th and 90th percentile points were 20 and 40 dB SPL for the 5-month-olds and 20 and 30 dB SPL for the 6- to 18-month-olds. Compared to thresholds obtained by BOA for the same ages (from Thompson & Weber, 1974), the VRA thresholds are lower. But of far greater importance is the reduced variability of response associated with the VRA procedure. For infants 6 months old and above, the range between the 10th and 90th percentile is reduced from the 45 to 50 dB reported for BOA to 10 dB (or one measurement step) for VRA.

Of further interest, from the point of view of clinical applicability, a total of 94 infants was tested to complete the sample reported. The data

FIGURE 1-12
Cumulative mean head-turn responses in blocks of stimulus trials as a function of reinforcement condition - infants 5 to 6 months of age (N = 20) (From J. M. Moore, W. R. Wilson, and G. Thompson, 1977.)

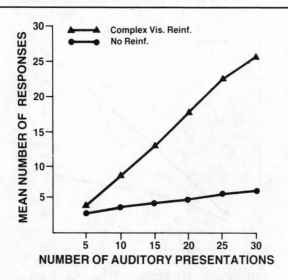

of three infants were not considered because of more than one false-positive response during the control intervals. (The average number of control intervals was 4.6 and the average number of false-positive responses was .37.) All but one infant 6 months of age and older yielded thresholds in one visit, with the exception requiring two visits. The clinical implications of this study are substantial: (1) thresholds obtained from infants do not vary dramatically as a function of age and are elevated only slightly from those obtained from adults using the same test protocol; (2) even more importantly, the range of thresholds for the population of presumed normal-hearing infants was very small, indicating that the values obtained can serve a usable function as clinical norms— a finding in direct contrast to the very wide dispersion demonstrated for BOA procedures; and (3) the procedure is economical of time and highly applicable to infants 6 months of age and older.

Whereas the above study used a broad-band signal, Wilson and Moore (1978) investigated the use of VRA with pure-tone stimuli in a soundfield. Two groups of 15 normally developing infant subjects—6 to 7 months of

FIGURE 1-13
Cumulative mean head-turn responses in blocks of stimulus trials as a function of reinforcement condition - infants 4 months of age (N = 20) (From J. M. Moore, W. R. Wilson, and G. Thompson, 1977.)

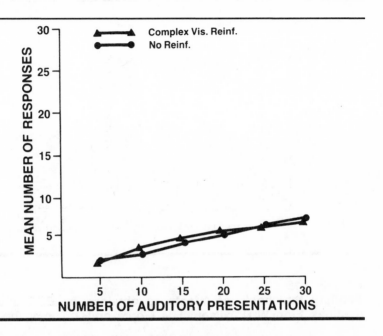

age and 12 to 13 months of age—were selected by the same criteria as in our previous studies. Pure tones of 500, 1000, and 4000 Hz with a 5% warble served as the auditory stimuli. (This study also included an earphone condition, which is described later in this chapter—the order of the soundfield and earphone conditions was counterbalanced.) Threshold measurement involved the same protocol described previously. Figure 1-16 provides the pure-tone soundfield thresholds for the two age groups of infants. As is apparent, thresholds do not vary systematically as a function of age, at least, given the 10-dB step size used in this experiment. The results obtained for the two groups of infants were collapsed and compared to a group (N = 10) of young adults, tested with the same protocol and step size, as shown in Figure 1-17. The difference in obtained thresholds is from 5 to 12 dB, depending on frequency, with the range of responses similar between the two groups. This study demonstrates that a pure-tone signal can be used successfully with infants and that the obtained thresholds do not vary dramatically from those of adults. The differences between these findings and those of earlier studies using BOA, with reference to

FIGURE 1-14
Infant head-turn responses as a function of reinforcement - single-subject design (From W. R. Wilson and J. M. Moore, 1978.)

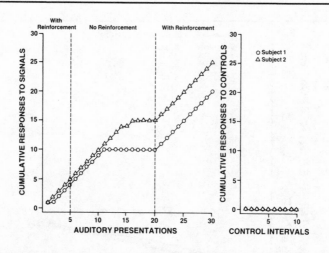

FIGURE 1-15
Auditory thresholds of infants as obtained by BOA and VRA methods (From W. R. Wilson, J. M. Moore, and G. Thompson, 1976.)

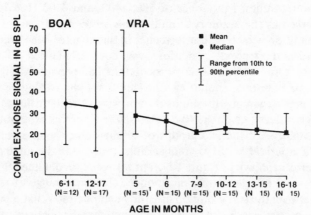

¹Six of the 15 did not complete test—data based on nine subjects

FIGURE 1-16
VRA PURETONE SOUNDFIELD THRESHOLDS — INFANT GROUPS
(From W. R. Wilson and J. M. Moore, 1978.)

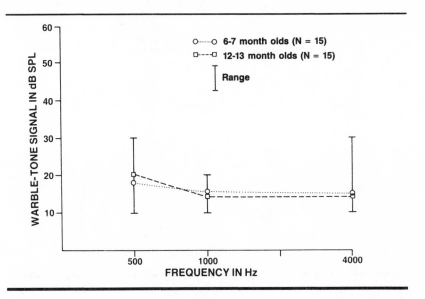

the use of pure-tone stimuli, demonstrate the important effect of methodology.

In a study similar to that of Wilson and Moore, accomplished in a different laboratory, Goldman (1979) also used VRA with infants 6 to 12 months of age. His test protocol was similar to that used by Wilson and Moore, including the use of control trials. Warbled (5%) pure-tone signals of 500, 1000, 2000, and 4000 Hz were presented in a soundfield test environment. Of the 29 infants studied, 23 were tested successfully at all four frequencies in one visit. For the remaining 6 subjects, 2 yielded thresholds at three test frequencies, 2 provided thresholds at two frequencies, 1 at a single frequency, and 1 gave no thresholds. The mean thresholds were 17 dB SPL at 500 Hz, 14 dB SPL at 1000 Hz, 17 dB SPL at 2000 Hz, and 15 dB SPL at 4000 Hz. Figure 1-18 provides a comparison of the Goldman (1979) and Wilson and Moore (1978) data, with both data sets plotted relative to young-adult thresholds for the same signal and protocol conditions. As can be noted, there is excellent agreement across studies accomplished in two different settings by two independent research groups, which lends support to the validity of the findings.

The above soundfield studies employed a test paradigm modeled on the clinical protocol used with adults and had as their main purpose the

FIGURE 1-17
VRA pure tone soundfield thresholds - infants and adults (From W. R. Wilson and J. M. Moore, 1978.)

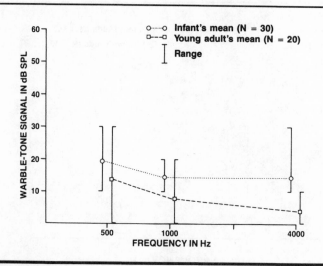

FIGURE 1-18
VRA pure tone soundfield threshold agreement across studies using a clinical protocol (W. R. Wilson and J. M. Moore, 1978.)

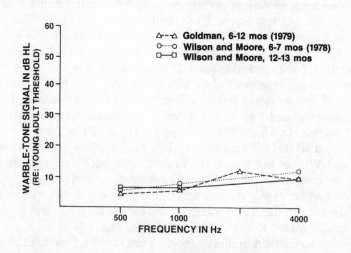

development of clinical procedures for infant auditory assessment. A modification of the VRA procedure described above has been developed by Trehub, Schneider, and colleagues (Schneider, Trehub, & Bull, 1979, 1980; Trehub, Schneider, & Endman, 1980) for studying basic auditory function in infants. Instead of using the fixed-interval discrimination task, as developed in our lab, they use a turn-left/turn-right localization task with unlimited duration stimulus intervals. Specifically, when the infant is looking directly ahead, a sound is presented from one of two loudspeakers located 45° to each side of the infant. The sound is terminated when the infant turns his or her head 45° to either side. If the head turn is correct—to the side of the sound—the response is reinforced. They describe the procedure as a two-alternative forced-choice signal detection task and use group data to plot psychometric functions for infant auditory thresholds.

Using half-octave and octave bands of noise as signals, Trehub, Schneider, and Endman (1980) and Schneider, Trehub, and Bull (1980) have used their procedure to chart infant hearing sensitivity from 200 through 19000 Hz. Figure 1-19 provides a comparison of the Wilson and Moore (1978) data, the Goldman (1979) data, and the Trehub, Schneider, and Endman (1980) data, as well as illustrating the overall pattern of the infant's sensitivity curve as developed by Trehub and colleagues. In comparing the infant results to those of adults in the same procedure, Trehub, Schneider, and Endman (1980) and Schneider, Trehub, and Bull (1980) report the greatest infant/adult differences in the low frequencies, with the infant thresholds equaling adult thresholds at the highest frequencies they studied. They postulate that the course of development in infant auditory sensitivity may be occurring primarily in the low frequencies. Several caveats should be considered relative to this interpretation, however. First, this presumes that the adult sensitivity has not declined in the high frequencies. Recent work by Fausti, Erickson, Frey, Rappaport, and Schechter (1981) with pure-tone frequencies through 20000 Hz suggests this is not true. Next, use of localization judgments for each signal presentation, as in the Trehub-Schneider procedure, may be problematic. Localization cues are frequency dependent, with interaural time differences predominating in the low frequencies and intensity differences in the high frequencies. Thus, results obtained with this procedure may reflect different infant abilities in the two areas of time and intensity resolution. It also should be noted that the use of a sound-field procedure that requires localization to both the right and left would be difficult for many clinical cases. For example, cases of unilateral loss or differences in sensitivity between the two ears would present difficulties.

Although not the focus of this chapter, interest in the issues surrounding the development of auditory sensitivity in infants and young children has resurfaced because of the methodological advances described in the

FIGURE 1-19
VRA soundfield thresholds across studies with differing methodologies (W. R. Wilson and J. M. Moore, 1978; T. M. Goldman, 1979; S. E. Trehub, B. A. Schneider, and M. Endman, 1980.)

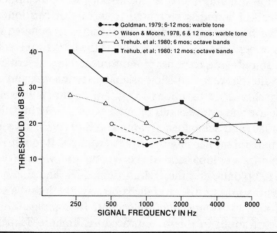

above studies. While not soundfield studies, several recent studies have re-addressed the same issues in children 4 to 12 years of age (Elliott & Katz, 1980; Maxon & Hochberg, 1982; Yoneshige & Elliott, 1981). Longitudinal study should now be possible and, when completed, will provide a better understanding of the development of auditory sensitivity.

Earphone Threshold Assessment

Since many clinical and research questions dealing with auditory sensitivity and perceptual abilities of infants demand individual ear data as well as greater signal specificity, Moore, Wilson, Lillis, and Talbott (1976) developed a headband/harness made of elastic and Velcro to hold a standard TDH-39 earphone and MX 41-AR cushion in place. Twenty infants between 6 and 8 months of age were selected as in the previous studies. The auditory signal was the same complex broad-band noise and the threshold protocol remained the same. Thresholds were obtained for both ears and soundfield—mean thresholds were 35 dB SPL for earphones and 28.5 dB SPL for the soundfield. Comparing the infant results to a small sample of young, normal-hearing adults, using the same signal and test protocol, the adult thresholds were approximately 10 dB better than the infant thresholds for each condition. The difference between the minimum audible field (MAF) and minimum audible pressure (MAP) values was the same—6 dB for both groups.

Wilson and Moore (1978) investigated the use of VRA with pure-tone stimuli under earphones. Two groups of normal infant subjects—6-7 months of age and 12-13 months—were selected with N = 15 in each group. The auditory stimuli were 5% warbled pure tones of 500, 1000, and 4000 Hz. The headband/harness made of elastic and Velcro, or a modified child's headset, held a standard TDH-39 earphone and MX 41-AR cushion in place on the left ear of each subject. Thresholds were determined using the same testing procedure as described above. On the average, two 15-minute sessions were required to obtain thresholds for the three pure-tone stimuli. Average thresholds were approximately 33 dB SPL at 500 Hz and approximately 24 dB SPL at 1000 and 4000 Hz. Figure 1-20 displays the results—at 1000 and 4000 Hz, no systematic threshold differences between the two age groups are observed. At 500 Hz, the younger infants are set apart from the older infants with poorer mean thresholds. Figure 1-21 groups the infant data and provides a comparison with a group of normal-hearing young adults run under the same conditions, including the 10 dB-step size. Whereas the infant/adult soundfield differences were 5 dB at 500 Hz and 12 dB at 4000 Hz in the same study, the infant/adult earphone differences were on the order of 16 dB at 500 Hz and 11 dB at 4000 Hz. Likewise, a comparison of the threshold curves in the sound-field condition (Figure 1-17) as compared to the threshold curves in the earphone condition (Figure 1-21) demonstrates an exaggerated rise in the low frequencies for the infant earphone condition. These findings have led us to question the possible effect of leakage around the earphone cushion as one cause of the elevated low-frequency earphone thresholds for the infants. A study in our lab currently is investigating these issues.

Nozza (1981), as a part of a study on critical ratios in infants, used a computer-controlled adaptive procedure to develop auditory thresholds in quiet and in noise. His procedure employed a 5-dB-step size with threshold defined as the mean of the intensity levels of the last eight turn-around points. Of interest here is the fact that the infants were able to accomplish this psychophysical procedure and yielded pure-tone thresholds in quiet of 19 dB at 1000 Hz and 15 dB at 4000 Hz under earphones. Nozza's results, accomplished in the same lab, may be compared to the Wilson and Moore earphone data using the clinical test paradigm (Figure 1-22). As is apparent, the use of the 5-dB-step size and the adaptive procedure reduces the thresholds by approximately 5 to 9 dB, as contrasted to those obtained with the 10-dB-step size and clinical procedure. One other factor, which

FIGURE 1-20
VRA pure tone earphone thresholds - infant groups (W. R. Wilson and J. M. Moore, 1978.)

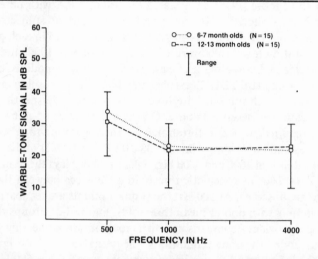

FIGURE 1-21
VRA pure tone earphone thresholds - infants and adults (From W. R. Wilson and J. M. Moore, 1978.)

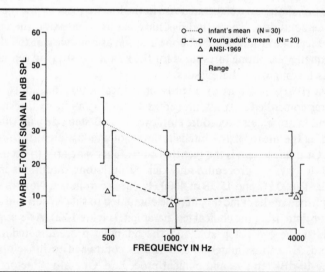

FIGURE 1-22
Comparison of VRA pure tone earphone thresholds as a function of test protocol (From W. R. Wilson and J. M. Moore, 1978; R. J. Nozza, 1981.)

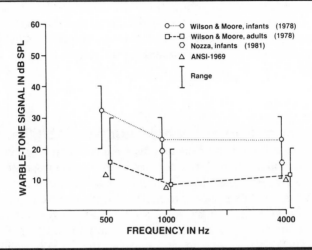

also may account for some of the difference, is that Nozza used an impedance screen in addition to the oral history/screen used by Wilson and Moore, and excluded any infants with negative middle-ear pressure in excess of -100 mm H_2O at the time of the test.

Throughout the discussions of the recent studies of auditory thresholds of infants, we have provided comparisons between adult and infant results. The reasons for the comparisons are two-fold. First, as noted above, an underlying theme in this literature is an interest in understanding the developmental course of auditory sensitivity. Second, the clinician needs to know the adult/infant threshold relationships in terms of assignment of "normal" threshold to obtained results as a function of age. Specific to this point, however, is the important fact that although the studies reported provide very tight groupings of obtained threshold values, caution must be exercised in generalizing these values to other clinics. Differences in signal, soundfield test environments, and VRA test protocol may lead to differences in individual clinic normative values. Each clinic should see a small sample of normally developing infants to establish normative data for that setting. The sample need not be large, based on the findings that infant dispersion data in these procedures are equal to that of young adults in the same procedures.

Finally, we do not take the infant/adult differences to indicate that infants' thresholds are *necessarily* less sensitive than adults'. The task expected of the infant involves responding to a low-level signal while being visually distracted with toys, in order to maintain the infant's attention toward a midline position. It is quite possible that a slightly higher level signal is required to overcome the attention directed toward visual stimulation as the infant is being "entertained" during the test procedure. No such visual distraction exists for adult testing. This question should be amenable to experimental manipulation and would be a fruitful area for further investigation.

Assessment of Suprathreshold Auditory Abilities

The VRA test procedure is an operant discrimination paradigm in which detection of a change in signal state coupled with a correct response allows reinforcement. Whereas the VRA threshold task involves detection of the presence or absence of signal, suprathreshold tasks involve detection of a change in signal. Initial work involving suprathreshold stimulation has been reported in the area of speech-sound discrimination. Eilers, Wilson, and Moore (1977) developed a procedure called the Visually Reinforced Infant Speech Discrimination (VRISD) paradigm to study developmental changes in discrimination as a function of age. All details of the VRA paradigm remained the same, except that one syllable of a recorded contrastive pair was presented in a repetition rate of one syllable per second at 50 dB SPL. While the infant was entertained at midline, the syllable was changed during a 4-second interval, with the temporal pattern of repetitions held constant. The infant was reinforced for a head turn to the change in signal by the activation of an animated toy. Initially, the *figure* (change) stimulus was presented at a higher intensity than the *ground* (background) stimulus. Once the infant had demonstrated responses to the intensity and/or speech-sound difference, the intensities were equated. Each infant was then presented with three change and three control (no-change) trials; to reach significance, the infant had to respond appropriately five out of six times.

Three studies using the VRISD procedure (Eilers, Gavin, & Wilson, 1979; Eilers, Wilson, & Moore, 1977, 1979) have shown that a high percentage of infants 6 to 14 months of age can be tested for discrimination of subtle speech contrasts. Furthermore, it has been demonstrated that the VRISD paradigm can provide data on individual infants on a repeated basis, in order to obtain information concerning discrimination of a variety of contrasts over time. Some infants have been tested on as many as 10 speech contrasts in as few as three 20-minute sessions. Since the original description of the VRISD procedure (Eilers, Wilson, & Moore, 1977), a number of researchers have used variations of the procedure to study different questions in the area of infant speech perception—for current reviews see Kuhl (1980) or Aslin, Pisoni, and Jusczyk (1983). Although the primary focus of this work, to date, has been on theoretical issues in the area of infant speech perception, the possibilities for applying this procedure to disordered populations are exciting. For example, since this discrimination procedure does not require receptive language abilities, as other tests of auditory discrimination for children do, testing of discrimination function can occur at a very early age. Further, as more information about the discrimination abilities of normal infants becomes available, there will exist a normative guide against which to compare performance of developmentally delayed youngsters. Resnick, Bookstein, and Talkin (1982) have described the results of preliminary work in this direction.

Diefendorf (1981) made use of the basic VRISD paradigm to study binaural fusion with infants 6- to 8-months old. Binaural fusion is the capacity of the auditory system to integrate separate inputs to the two ears into a single auditory percept. When the two ears are stimulated by dichotic speech signals (signals differing with respect to each other in one or more signal parameters), a listener perceives one central image and is incapable of separating the individual speech signals. When the left or right ear only is stimulated, no centrally fused subjective image is formed. Diefendorf (1981) used two computer-generated speech-like vowels made up of a high and low passband each. The four waveforms (two vowels × two passbands) could be instrumentally presented with the low passband of vowel 1 combined with the high passband of either vowel 1 or vowel 2. Likewise, the low passband of vowel 2 could be combined with the high passband of either vowel 2 or vowel 1. The resultant four signals could be presented in diotic or dichotic mix. If one of the "vowel" sounds was discriminated from the second "vowel" sound, four possible explanations could account for this behavior. First, it is possible that the dichotic presentations fused, and the infant discriminated one vowel sound from the other vowel sound, diotic or dichotic. A second, and equally plausible, explanation is that the infants simply memorized which individual vowel sounds were reinforced and which were not. With only four items, an infant might remember which two vowel sounds were reinforced and which two were not. Finally, it is possible that the infants discriminated the two vowels by paying attention to either the high or the low pitch of the two-formant vowel. Since the high and low formant of each vowel have a different pitch, then, by simply listening to or perceiving the high or low pitch of each vowel, the infant could discriminate one from the other, regardless of whether the vowel was presented diotically or dichotically. Therefore, four experiments were run with four separate groups of infants and four different signal combinations to address each of the possible outcomes: (1) binaural fusion; (2) memory; (3) high-formant discrimination; and (4) low-formant discrimination.

The results showed that the infants in the fusion group maintained a perception of the two vowels regardless of whether or not the presentation was diotic or dichotic. The other infants were not able to resolve the task by memorizing two of four stimuli or by discriminating on the basis of low- or high-formant information only. Thus, the results of this study suggest that 6- to 8-month-old infants demonstrate fusion of auditory information in the central auditory system.

The literature reports that binaural fusion has been utilized as a test of central auditory function with children as young as 5 years of age (Willeford, 1977). Additionally, Willeford suggested that this ability seems to be age related, showing a "maturational pattern" from ages 5 through 9. The mean scores on Willeford's norms do improve with age. However, the wide dispersion of scores, at any single age, raises questions about task variables as contrasted to developmental or maturational factors in binaural fusion. The data from Diefendorf (1981) would suggest that binaural fusion may not be strongly age related, since infants at 6 months of age demonstrated success on a binaural fusion task. In most previous fusion tasks, words or sentences have been used as stimuli. With adults and older children, this may not affect the outcome. However, with young children, one would expect language to be a critical factor. In addition, the clinical populations of interest in many cases are those with demonstrated language/learning difficulties. Instructions, memory, and response task can also play a role in the outcome of a binaural fusion task. If the task requires oral and/or written instruction, its use will again be restricted in terms of the age and language level of persons for whom it will be appropriate. Memory and response task interact in that certain responses (e.g., "point to the picture") place additional memory constraints on the task, as well as introducing visual-motor components to the procedure. we feel that the approach employed in the VRISD procedure overcomes many of these problems and can be applied to other studies of central auditory function in normals and, eventually, in the clinic.

Three studies (Bull, Schneider, & Trehub, 1981; Nozza, 1981; Trehub, Bull, & Schneider, 1981) have explored the topic of masking with infants using head-turn procedures. Masking studies not only provide information relative to the effect of noise (or other masking signals) on thresholds, but also on the basic frequency selectivity of the ear. Masking is a consequence of the ear's limited frequency selectivity—as the energy in a masking stimulus approaches a test stimulus in frequency, there is an increase in the masking effect. Bull, Schneider, and Trehub (1981) and Trehub, Schneider, and Bull (1981) used the turn-right/turn-left unlimited-response-interval procedure to study the effects of broad-band noise on a 4000-Hz center frequency octave band (Bull et al.) and on a speech phrase (Trehub et al.). Subjects were 6- , 12- , 18- , and 24-month-old infants and adults. Increases in masking levels produced comparable threshold shifts for all age groups. Nozza (1981), using the fixed-interval unidirection head-turn procedure with 6- and 12-month-old infants and adults, found similar results for pure-tone stimuli and a broad-band masker. Collectively these studies suggest that the use of a masking signal in a clinical paradigm should produce similar results in infants and adults. In terms of frequency selectivity, Nozza's work demonstrated that the critical ratios—inferred auditory-filter-bandwidth estimates—are proportional for all ages. The actual critical ratios of infants are larger than those of adults. However, the infant/adult difference results from elevated infant thresholds in the detection-in-noise condition. The reader will recall a systematic infant/adult difference in threshold estimates. Nozza argues that the consistent relationship between infant and adult thresholds across studies may point to the effect of attention/motivational factors. His work is important in providing initial information in the area of frequency selectivity in infants and suggests that more direct measures such as band-limiting experiments may be possible.

In the area of frequency discrimination, Olsho, Schoon, Sakai, Turpin, and Sperduto (1982) used the fixed-interval unidirection head-turn procedure with 5- to 8-month-old infants. The signal was a repeating background tone (1000, 2000, and 3000 Hz pure tones) which was contrasted to a variable target tone. Their results suggested that infants could detect a two-percent change in frequency, whereas adults detected changes of one percent or less. The infant data showed considerable variability, however. Continued work in the area of frequency and intensity discrimination is underway in several labs at present. As the results of these normative studies describe the developmental course in each area, clinical applications should become possible.

Application to Developmentally Disabled Populations

Greenberg, Wilson, Moore, and Thompson (1978) investigated the effectiveness of VRA with infants and young children with Down's syndrome. There were 41 subjects between 6 months and 6 years of age. Twenty-five of the subjects were also administered the *Bayley Scales of Infant Development (BSID)*. VRA soundfield threshold test procedures, as previously described, were used. Each subject was required to respond to two out of three presentations (complex noise) at either a 50 or 70 dB SPL conditioning level. If a subject failed to satisfy this initial conditioning criterion, an attempt was made to teach the turning response by pairing the auditory and visual stimulus. If consistent responses occurred within a maximum of 10 teaching trials, the original test procedure was again attempted. Results were as follows: (1) 28 (68%) of the subjects spontaneously oriented toward the source of the auditory stimulus; (2) only a few of the subjects who did not initially orient could be taught to respond; (3) of the children who initially oriented or were taught to respond, thresholds were obtained on a large number (81%) in one visit; and (4) a systematic relationship was demonstrated between consistency of response using the VRA technique and *BSID* Mental Age Equivalent, with 10 months being the critical age for determining the potential success of the procedure. The threshold values ranged from 30-60 dB SPL with a mean of 38.4 dB SPL. These results can be compared to those obtained on 75 normal infants between 6 and 18 months of age (Wilson, Moore, & Thompson, 1976), whose thresholds ranged from 10-40 dB SPL with a mean of 22.5 dB SPL.

Interpretation of these threshold data as fundamental indicators of hearing sensitivity is complicated by the possibility that some subjects may have been experiencing mild middle ear involvement at the time of testing. Both the Greenberg, Wilson, Moore, and Thompson (1978) and Wilson, Moore, and Thompson (1976) studies attempted to minimize the effects of middle ear involvement through subject selection procedures. These included no cold on the test day and no recent history of middle ear problems. Tympanometry results were not reported, however, which leaves open the possibility that the average threshold data for the subjects with Down's syndrome, in particular, may have been slightly inflated above true sensorineural hearing status, since this population has been shown to have a high incidence of middle ear involvement (Balkany, Downs, Jafek, & Krajicek, 1979; Brooks, Wooley, & Kanjilal, 1972; Schwartz & Schwartz, 1978).

In regard to the age at which children with Down's syndrome can be satisfactorily tested with VRA, the Greenberg, Wilson, Moore, and Thompson study (1978) suggested that a mental-age equivalent (i.e., a functioning level) of 10 months was required. A follow-up study (Thompson, Wilson, and Moore, 1979) supported this finding. In view of this, it is of interest that in recent months, we have seen clinically a few infants with Down's syndrome who have performed VRA satisfactorily at a *chronological* age of approximately 10 months. Each of these particular infants demonstrated hearing thresholds at about 20 dB HL, had normal tympanograms, had *never* experienced middle ear involvement (parental report) and were involved in a formal infant-stimulation program in an educational setting. One hesitates to place undue emphasis on a few clinical cases; still, it is tempting to speculate on the developmental advantage that may accrue to infants with Down's syndrome who have been free of middle ear involvement since birth and who have been involved in programs designed to maximize communication skills.

Refinement of VRA Test Paradigm

Over the past years, our research using the visual reinforcement paradigm has incorporated a number of changes designed to tighten experimental controls and facilitate test administration. The first of these involved design of a logic circuit to allow greater control during testing. A control box was designed which consisted of a simple AND-Gate circuit. The presentation of an auditory stimulus starts an adjustable timer which is used to define the response interval—usually set at 4 seconds. If the infant responds correctly during the 4-second period, and if both examiners independently vote that a response occurred, the visual reinforcer is automatically activated for a preselected duration—usually 2 or 3 seconds. If one or both examiners vote after the response-interval timer has elapsed, indicating the infant responded after the 4-second response period, the visual reinforcer will not be activated. Also, if only one examiner votes, even if the timer is still on, the reinforcer will not be activated. If a single examiner is testing, a shorting plug can be substituted for the test-room vote button and the logic features are still operational. If the vote-logic circuit is not desired, as is the case when first conditioning the infants to respond, a manual override system is available which allows the examiner to activate the visual reinforcer by a single button push. A detailed description of the equipment used in the VRA test paradigm is available (Wilson, Lee, Owen, & Moore, 1976). The vote-logic circuit provides a precise definition of the response interval for both signal presentation and control trials. Likewise, the determination of whether or not reinforcement should be provided is based on the positive judgment of both examiners that a head turn has occurred during the response interval. Finally, since the response-interval timer is automatically activated at signal onset and reinforcement is automatically controlled, the task is made easier for the examiner and his or her full attention can be devoted to observing the infant.

The second area of improvement in the VRA paradigm dealt with the test-room examiner. The role of this individual is crucial to the success of the VRA procedure. Yet the possibility exists that his or her behavior, in terms of manipulation of objects during signal-presentation intervals and control intervals, could significantly influence the outcome of the test. Likewise, if signal presentation always occurred when the child was in an optimum response state, and control intervals always occurred when the infant was highly interested and actively involved with the toys and test-room examiner, the effectiveness of the control intervals in defining false-positive response rates would be minimized. To control these potential sources of bias, several refinements in the VRA test paradigm were introduced. The test-room examiner wears earphones and is alerted by a tone that a judgment period is occurring. During soundfield testing, a masking signal is presented so that he or she cannot hear the auditory signal presentations, thereby removing that potential source of bias. The possible problem with determination of signal presentation versus control interval is handled by having the test-room examiner indicate when the infant is in a response-ready state. Then, the control-room examiner initiates either a signal presentation or a control interval, working from a prerandomized trial schedule, or by use of a probability generator built into the equipment which automatically selects whether a control interval or an auditory stimulus is presented. A small computer may also be used for handling the logic needs as well as controlling the signal.

A third general area of modification of the VRA paradigm dealt with the visual reinforcer. We observed that some of the infants stared or continued to glance at the visual reinforcer (i.e., toy animal) during the test session. This made testing more difficult because the examiner had to get the infant actively involved with toys in order to return him or her to a midline position. If the individual and/or activities become more interesting than the reinforcer, the infant might not respond. Also, we reasoned that if the animated toy was seen only during reinforcement periods following a correct response, this might increase the strength of the visual reinforcer. It was decided to try an enclosure made of dark, smoked plexiglass with two small 40-watt light bulbs connected on the inside in front of the toy animal. When the reinforcer is not activated, the enclosure appears as a nondescript black box. When activated, the box is illuminated, revealing the animated toy.

A final observation is related to choice of reinforcers. Although seemingly a trivial matter, we have found that it is advantageous to have different animated toys wired so that they may be substituted easily during a test session. We also have arranged two reinforcers in a stacked fashion within a single enclosure, each of which is activated on a .5 random probability (probability generator). In some clinical situations, when a return visit by the infant would be difficult for logistical reasons, it is possible to extend the duration of the session by either of these approaches.

Epilogue

Almost four decades ago, Ewing and Ewing (1944) commented, "There is an urgent need to study further and more critically methods of testing hearing in young children." Over the years, considerable progress has been made in this direction, particularly with regard to the measurement of hearing sensitivity. In many respects, though, their comment continues to be relevant as it applies generally to the study of infant auditory perception. It will be of interest to evaluate the course of events over the next 40 years for those fortunate ones among us in a position to do so.

Acknowledgment

The research accomplished at the Child Development and Mental Retardation Center, University of Washington, has been supported in part by grants from The Deafness Research Foundation; the National Foundation—March of Dimes; Maternal and Child Health Services; and National Institute of Child Health and Human Development. The authors express their appreciation to Linda Hesketh for her assistance in preparation of the manuscript.

Note

Audiometric thresholds and intensity levels are reported in dB SPL, since no standard exists for converting these values into comparable HL. For comparative purposes, the modal threshold of normal hearing young-adult listeners was 20 dB SPL, with a range of 10 dB SPL to 20 dB SPL, under the same signal and measurement-step conditions.

References

Aslin, R.N., Pisoni, D.B., & Jusczyk, P.W. Auditory development and speech perception in infancy. In M.M. Haith & J.J. Campos (Eds.), *Infancy and the biology of development.* New York, Wiley & Sons, 1983.

Balkany, T., Downs, M.P., Jafek, B.W., & Krajicek, M.J. Hearing loss in Down's syndrome. *Clinical Pediatrics*, 1979, *18*, 116-118.

Brooks, D.N., Wooley, H., & Kanjilal, G.C. Hearing loss and middle ear disorders in patients with Down's syndrome (mongolism). *Journal of Mental Deficiency Research*, 1972, *16*, 21-29.

Bull, D., Schneider, B.A., & Trehub, S.E. The masking of octave-band noise by broad-spectrum noise: A comparison of infant and adult thresholds. *Perception and Psychophysics*, 1981, *30*, 101-106.

Diefendorf, A.O. *An investigation of one aspect of central auditory function in an infant popula-tion utilizing a binaural resynthesis (fusion) task.* Unpublished doctoral dissertation, University of Washington, 1981.

Downs, M.P., & Sterritt, G.M. A guide to newborn and infant hearing screening programs. *Archives of Otolaryngology,* 1967, *85,* 15-22.

Eilers, R.E. Development of phonology. In F.D. Minifie & L.L. Lloyd (Eds.), *Communicative and cognitive abilities—Early behavioral assessment.* Baltimore: University Park Press, 1978.

Eilers, R.E., Gavin, W., & Wilson, W.R. Linguistic experience and phonemic perception in infancy: A cross-linguistic study. *Child Development,* 1979, *50,* 14-18.

Eilers, R.E., Wilson, W.R., & Moore J.M. Developmental changes in speech discrimination in infants. *Journal of Speech and Hearing Research,* 1977, *20,* 766-780.

Eilers, R.E., Wilson, W.R., & Moore, J.M. Speech discrimination in the language-innocent and the language-wise: A study in the perception of voice onset time. *Journal of Child Language,* 1979, *6,* 1-18.

Eisele, W.A., Berry, R.C., & Shriner, T.H. Infant sucking response patterns as a conjugate function of changes in the sound pressure level of auditory stimuli. *Journal of Speech and Hearing Research,* 1975, *18,* 296-307.

Eisenberg, R.B. *Auditory competence in early life—The roots of communicative behavior.* Baltimore: University Park Press, 1976.

Elliott, L.L., & Katz, D.R. Children's pure-tone detection. *Journal of the Acoustical Society of America,* 1980, *67,* 343-344.

Ewing, I.R., & Ewing, A.W.G. The ascertainment of deafness in infancy and early childhood. *Journal of Laryngology and Otology,* 1944, *59,* 309-333.

Fausti, S. A., Erickson, D. A., Frey, R. H., Rappaport, B. Z. & Schechter, M. A. The effects of noise upon human hearing sensitivity from 8000 to 20000 Hz. *Journal of the Acoustical Society of America,* 1981, *69,* 1343-1349.

Field, J., DiFranco, D., Dodwell, P., & Muir, D. Auditory-visual coordination in two and one-half-month-old infants. *Infant Behaviour and Development,* 1979, *2,* 113-122.

Field, J., Muir, D., Pilon, R., Sinclair, M., & Dodwell, P. Infants' orientation to lateral sounds from birth to three months. *Child Development,* 1980, *51,* 295-298.

Friedlander, B. Automated playtest systems for evaluating infant's and young children's selec-tive listening to natural sounds and language. Scientific exhibit presented at the American Speech and Hearing Association Convention, Chicago, 1969.

Friedlander, B.Z. Receptive language development in infancy: Issues and problems. *Merrill-Palmer Quarterly,* 1970, *16,* 7-51.

Gans, D.P., & Flexer, C. Observer bias in the hearing testing of profoundly involved multip-ly handicapped children. *Ear and Hearing,* 1982, *3,* 309-313.

Goldman, T.M. Response of infants to warble-tone signals presented in soundfield using visual reinforcement audiometry. Master's thesis, University of Cincinnati, 1979.

Goldstein, R., & Tait, C. Critique of neonatal hearing evaluation. *Journal of Speech and Hear-ing Disorders,* 1971, *36,* 3-18.

Greenberg, D.B., Wilson, W.R., Moore, J.M., & Thompson, G. Visual reinforcement audiometry (VRA) with young Down's syndrome children. *Journal of Speech and Hearing Disorders,* 1978, *43,* 448-458.

Haug, O., Baccaro, P., & Guilford, F.R. A pure-tone audiogram on the infant: The PIWI technique. *Archives of Otolaryngology,* 1967, *86,* 435-440.

Hoversten, G., & Moncur J. Stimuli and intensity factors in testing infants. *Journal of Speech and Hearing Research,* 1969, *12,* 687-702.

Kuhl, P.K. Infant speech perception: Reviewing data on auditory category formation. In P. Levinson & C. Sloan (Eds.), *Auditory processing and language: Clinical and research perspec-tives.* New York: Grune & Stratton, 1980.

Liden, G., & Kankkunen, A. Visual reinforcement audiometry. *Acta Oto-laryngologica*, 1969, *67*, 281-292.

Ling D., Ling, A.H., & Doehring, D.G. Stimulus response and observer variables in the auditory screening of newborn infants. *Journal of Speech and Hearing Research*, 1970, *13*, 9-18.

Maxon, A.B., & Hochberg, I. Development of psychoacoustic behavior: Sensitivity and discrimination. *Ear and Hearing*, 1982, *3*, 301-308.

Moncur, J.P. Judge reliability in infant testing. *Journal of Speech and Hearing Disorders.* 1968, *11*, 348-357.

Moore, J.M., Thompson, G., & Thompson, M. Auditory localization of infants as a function of reinforcement conditions. *Journal of Speech and Hearing Disorders*, 1975, *40*, 29-34.

Moore, J.M., Wilson, W.R., Lillis, K.E., & Talbott, S.A. Earphone audiometry thresholds of infants utilizing visual reinforcement audiometry (VRA). Paper presented at the American Speech and Hearing Association Convention, Houston, 1976.

Moore, J.M., Wilson, W.R., & Thompson, G. Visual reinforcement of head-turn responses in infants under 12 months of age. *Journal of Speech and Hearing Disorders*, 1977, *42*, 328-334.

Morse, P.A. Infant speech perception: Origins, processes, and *alpha centauri.* In F.D. Minifie & L.L. Lloyd (Eds.), *Communicative and cognitive abilities—Early behavioral assessment.* Baltimore: University Park Press, 1978.

Motta, G., Facchini, G.M., & D'Auria, E. Objective conditioned-reflex audiometry in children. *Acta Oto-Laryngologica*, Suppl. 273, 1970, 1-49.

Muir, D., Abraham, W., Forbes, B., & Harris, L. The ontogenesis of an auditory localization response from birth to four months of age. *Canadian Journal of Psychology*, 1979, *33*, 320-333.

Muir, D., & Field, J. Newborn infants orient to sounds. *Child Development*, 1979, *50*, 431-436.

Northern, J.L., & Downs M.P. *Hearing in children.* Baltimore: Williams & Wilkins, 1978.

Nozza, R.J. *Detection of pure tones in quiet and in noise by infants and adults.* Unpublished doctoral dissertation, University of Washington, 1981.

Olsho, L.W., Schoon, C., Sakai, R., Turpin, R., & Sperduto, V. Preliminary data on frequency discrimination in infancy. *Journal of the Acoustical Society of America*, 1982, *71*, 509-511.

Resnick, S.B., Bookstein, E.W., & Talkin, D. Clinical measurement of nonsense syllable discrimination in infants. Paper presented at the American Speech-Language-Hearing Association Convention, Toronto, 1982.

Schneider, B.A., Trehub, S.E., & Bull, D. The development of basic auditory processes in infants. *Canadian Journal of Psychology*, 1979, *33*, 306-319.

Schneider, B.A., Trehub, S.E., & Bull, D. High-frequency sensitivity in infants. *Science*, 1980, *207*, 1003-1004.

Schwartz, D.M., & Schwartz, R.H. Acoustic impedance and otoscopic findings in young children with Down's syndrome. *Archives of Otolaryngology*, 1978, *104*, 652-656.

Suzuki, T., & Ogiba, Y. A technique of pure-tone audiometry for children under three years of age: Conditioned orientation reflex (COR) audiometry. *Revue de Laryngologie, Otologie, Rhinologie*, 1960, *81*, 33-45.

Suzuki, T., & Ogiba, Y. Conditioned orientation reflex audiometry. *Archives of Otolaryngology*, 1961, *74*, 192-198.

Suzuki, T., & Sato, I. Free field startle response audiometry. *Annals of Otology, Rhinology and Laryngology*, 1961, *70*, 998-1007.

Sweitzer, R.S. Audiologic evaluation of the infant and young child. In B.F. Jaffe (Ed.). *Hearing loss in children.* Baltimore: University Park Press, 1977.

Thompson, G., & Weber, B.A. Responses of infants and young children to behavior observation audiometry (BOA). *Journal of Speech and Hearing Disorders*, 1974, *39*, 140-147.

Thompson, G., Wilson, W.R., & Moore, J.M. Application of visual reinforcement audiometry (VRA) to low-functioning children. *Journal of Speech and Hearing Disorders,* 1979, *44,* 80-90.

Thompson, M., & Thompson, G. Response of infants and young children as a function of auditory stimuli and test methods. *Journal of Speech and Hearing Research,* 1972, *15,* 699-707.

Trehub, S.E., Bull, D., & Schneider, B.A. Infants' detection of speech and noise. *Journal of Speech and Hearing Research,* 1981, *24,* 202-206.

Trehub, S.E., Schneider, B.A., & Bull, D. Effect of reinforcement on infants' performance in an auditory detection task. *Developmental Psychology,* 1981, *17,* 872-877.

Trehub, S.E., Schneider, B.A., & Endman, M. Developmental changes in infants' sensitivity to octave-band noises. *Journal of Experimental Child Psychology,* 1980, *29,* 282-293.

Weber, B.A. Validation of observer judgments in behavioral observation audiometry. *Journal of Speech and Hearing Disorders,* 1969, *34,* 350-355.

Weber, B.A. Comparison of two approaches to behavioral observation audiometry. *Journal of Speech and Hearing Research,* 1970, *13,* 823-825.

Willeford, J.A. Assessing central auditory behavior in children: A test battery approach. In R.W. Keith (Ed.), *Central auditory dysfunction.* New York: Grune & Stratton, 1977.

Wilson, W.R., Lee, K., Owen, G., & Moore, J.M. Instrumentation for operant infant auditory assessment. Seattle: Child Development and Mental Retardation Center, 1976.

Wilson, W.R., & Moore, J.M. Pure-tone earphone thresholds of infants utilizing visual reinforcement audiometry (VRA). Paper presented at the American Speech and Hearing Association Convention, San Francisco, 1978.

Wilson, W.R., Moore, J.M., & Thompson, G. Sound-field auditory thresholds of infants utilizing visual reinforcement audiometry (VRA). Paper presented at the American Speech and Hearing Association Convention, Houston, 1976.

Yoneshige, Y., & Elliott, L.L. Pure-tone sensitivity and ear canal pressure at threshold in children and adults. *Journal of the Acoustical Society of America,* 1981, *70,* 1272-1276.

Daniel J. Orchik
Karla S. MacKimmie

Immittance Audiometry

In summarizing his early clinical experience with immittance audiometry, Jerger (1970) stated that "quite frankly we wonder how we ever got along without it." Indeed, this procedure has stood the test of time and remains one of the most useful clinical tools in audiology, particularly in the evaluation of pediatric patients.

In pediatric audiology, immittance audiometry has been of particular utility in two general areas: the identification of middle ear disease and the identification of sensorineural hearing loss through acoustic reflex measures. In both areas, initial enthusiasm has been tempered somewhat by continuing research, but the usefulness of immittance audiometry has not been reduced. Rather, the informed clinician now utilizes immittance audiometry more effectively.

This chapter reviews the developments in both general areas mentioned above. In addition, some of the early work in immittance audiometry will also be reviewed to provide a needed perspective.

Immittance Audiometry: An Overview

The first clinical application of immittance audiometry is generally credited to Metz (1946), although the electroacoustic instruments in general clinical use today have evolved from the early work of Terkildsen and Scott-Nielsen (1960). The immittance battery, as currently employed, typically consists of three measures: tympanometry, static compliance, and acoustic reflex thresholds.

Tympanometry is a measurement of the relative change in compliance of the middle ear system as air pressure is varied in the external ear canal. Tympanograms, the graphic display of the tympanometric measurements, are generally classified in terms of the depth, shape, and point of middle ear pressure (Feldman, 1976, p. 119). One such classification scheme is shown in Figure 2-1. (Northern & Downs, 1974, p. 178). More elaborate systems have been developed, but all utilize the same basic parameters for interpretation (Orchik, Dunn, & McNutt, 1978; Paradise, Smith, & Bluestone, 1976).

Static compliance represents a measurement of the compliance of the middle ear system in its resting state. It is expressed in terms of a volume of air (in cm³) equivalent in compliance to that presented by the middle ear system. Static compliance is tested by making two equivalent volume measurements, one with a positive pressure of 200 mmH$_2$O at the tympanic membrane and the other with the tympanic membrane at its most compliant pressure point (Northern & Downs, 1978, p. 158).

The acoustic reflex threshold represents the minimum intensity that will result in a detectable reflexive contraction of the stapedial muscle. In most clinical applications of acoustic reflex threshold measurement, stimuli include pure tones at octave intervals from 500 through 4000 Hz. In addition, for specific applications, namely the prediction of sensorineural acuity, broad-band signals are also employed (Jerger, Burney, Mauldin, & Crump, 1974).

Immittance Audiometry in Middle Ear Disease

The most common cause of hearing loss in children is middle ear disease and by far the most common form of middle ear disease is otitis media and its associated complications (Goin, 1975). In fact, 90% of all ear problems in children are the result of some form of otitis media (McCandless, 1979). This disorder refers to the accumulation of fluid in the middle ear as a result of infection. Otitis media may be serous or suppurative, depending upon the infectious status of the middle ear fluid. The disease may also be chronic or acute depending upon the duration of the disease. Finally, it may be accompanied by complications such as tympanic membrane perforation and cholesteatoma.

In addition, the prevalence of this disorder has raised concern about the effect of the concomitant conductive hearing loss upon speech and

FIGURE 2-1
Classification of Tympanograms After Jerger (1970) (From *Hearing in Children* by J. Northern and M. Downs, 1974, Chapter 6: Copyright 1974 by Williams and Wilkins. Reprinted by permission.)

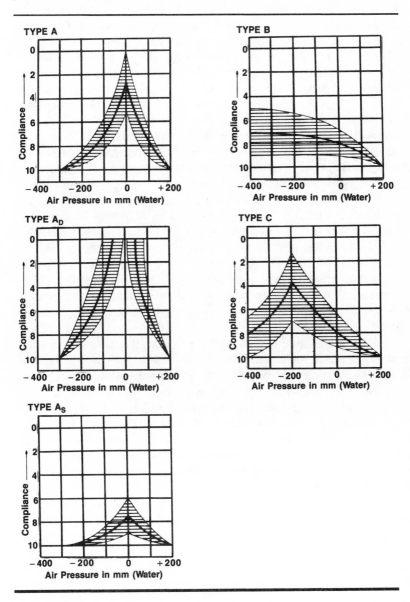

language development (Holm & Kunze, 1969; Kaplan, Fleshman, Bender, Baum, & Clark, 1973). Further, Brooks (1980) has recently suggested that recurrent or chronic middle ear disease in childhood may interact with the expected age-related hearing loss in the elderly, producing the need for amplification at a significantly earlier age.

Brooks (1968) was among the first to demonstrate the efficiency of using immittance audiometry in the detection of middle ear disease in children. Brooks observed that the primary effects of serous otitis media were a reduction in the depth of the tympanogram, which he termed the "gradient," and an associated decrease in static compliance.

Bluestone, Beery, and Paradise (1973) demonstrated the superiority of immittance testing over traditional pure-tone audiometry in the identification of middle-ear disease. In their investigation, the presence of serous otitis media was validated at myringotomy. Only tympanometry was used in immittance testing, along with pure-tone air conduction and bone conduction audiometry. In total, 84 children were examined. The presence of otitis media was found to be strongly related to tympanogram type. As shown in Figure 2-2, tympanograms characterized by reduced depth (types 4 and 5) were most likely to be found in ears with effusion. Perhaps more notable was the fact that of 34 cases with pure-tone averages better than 25 dB HTL (ANSI-69), 16 were found to have serous otitis media at myringotomy. All 16 cases demonstrated a type 4 or 5 tympanogram, and eight of these cases had pure tone averages of 15 dB HTL or better. Thus, Bluestone and his colleagues demonstrated the superiority of immittance measurement over pure-tone audiometry in the identification of middle ear disease in children.

Paradise, Smith, and Bluestone (1979) developed the classification system shown in Figure 2-3 in a study designed to further delineate the relationship between tympanometry and middle ear disease in children. In general, the results were consistent with previous reports in that tympanograms characterized by a rounded, shallow, or flat configuration were most commonly found in middle ear disorder. Cantekin, Bluestone, Fria, Stool, Beery, and Sabo (1980) confirmed these data in a study of 333 children employing the same system of classification for tympanometric data.

The relationship between degree of otitis media and tympanogram type was examined by Orchik, Dunn, and McNutt (1978). Tympanograms were classified using a system similar to that devised by Jerger (1970) and shown in Figure 2-4. Degree of otitis media was described in terms of the amount of middle ear effusion present at myringotomy. A total of 142 ears of 75 patients were examined, and the results suggested that when a type B tympanogram was found, there was approximately a 90% probability of significant middle ear effusion. Other tympanogram types were not efficient

FIGURE 2-2
Tympanograms and Findings at Myringotomy (From "Audiometry and Tympanometry in Relation to Middle Ear Effusion in Children" by C. Bluestone, Q. Beery, and J. Paradise, *Laryngoscope*, 1973, *83*, 594-604. Copyright 1973 by The Laryngoscope Company. Reprinted by permission.)

TYMPANOMETRIC PATTERN	NUMBER OF EARS		
	TOTAL	PRESENCE OF EFFUSION NO	YES
1 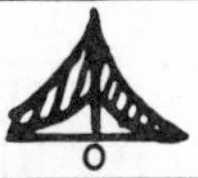	7	7	0
2 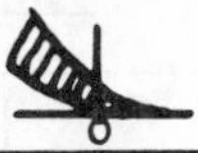	1	1	0
3 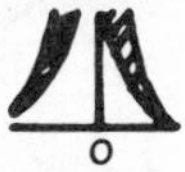	5	5	0
4 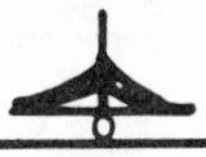	2	0	2
5 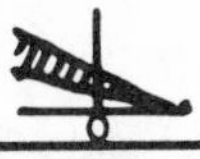	19	5	14
TOTAL EARS	34	18	16

predictors of serous otitis media. Renvall, Jarlstedt, and Holmquist (1980) reported similar data in a study of 103 Swedish children.

All of the preceding research has dealt only with tympanometry as opposed to the use of the complete immittance battery, which also includes static compliance and acoustic reflex testing. The relationship between otitis media and the immittance battery was examined by Orchik, Morff, and Dunn (1978). Data were obtained for 76 ears prior to myringotomy. The tympanometric data were similar to previous reports in that the type B tympanogram was associated with significant middle ear effusion in 90% of the ears presenting such a pattern.

Static compliance data were the least useful in detecting otitis media, while acoustic reflex data were similar in sensitivity to the tympanometric

FIGURE 2-3
Classification of Tympanograms Used by Paradise (From "Tympanometric Detection of Middle Ear Effusion in Infants and Young Children" by J. Paradise, D. Smith, and C. Bluestone, *Pediatrics*, 1976, *58*, 198-210. Copyright 1976 by The American Academy of Pediatrics. Reprinted by permission.)

Clinical Impedance Audiometry

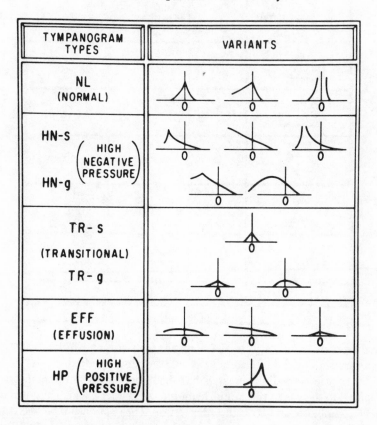

data. More important, perhaps, was the finding that the combined use of tympanometry and acoustic reflex testing may be superior to either measure alone in the identification of otitis media. As shown in Table 2-1, both the degree of false positive and false negative were reduced if both measures were employed (Orchik, Morff, & Dunn, 1978). Subsequent research has

FIGURE 2-4
Tympanometric Classifications Employed by Orchik (From "Tympanometry as a Predictor of Middle Ear Effusion" by D. Orchik, J. Dunn, and L. McNutt, *Archives of Otolaryngology*, *104*, 4-6. Copyright 1978 by the American Medical Association. Reprinted by permission.)

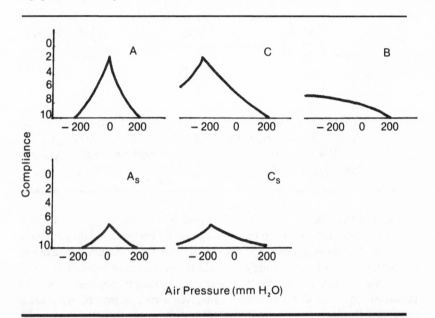

Air Pressure (mm H₂O)

supported the equivalent sensitivity of tympanometry and acoustic reflex testing, as well as the improved sensitivity offered by combining these two components of the immittance battery (Freyss, Narcy, Manac'h, & Toupet, 1980; Northern & Zarnoch, 1978).

From the preceding discussion, it is apparent that the immittance battery is extremely sensitive to the presence of middle ear disease in children. This fact, coupled with the previously mentioned concern about the effect of recurrent or chronic middle ear disease upon speech and language development, led to the widespread employment of immittance audiometry in pediatric hearing-screening programs. However, in more recent literature one can sense a kind of backlash against a perceived overuse of immittance audiometry in the identification of middle ear disease in children. This is particularly true where hearing conservation programs are concerned (Bluestone et al., 1980). A number of issues are involved in this controversy, including incidence, pathogenesis, and effective treatment for middle

Table 2-1
Comparison of False-Positive and False-Negative with use of Tympanometry and Acoustic Reflex Thresholds Alone or in Combination.

Rate	Tympanometry Alone	Acoustic Reflex Alone	Combined
False-positive (%)	18	22	10
False-negative (%)	10	10	0

NOTE: From Impedance Audiometry in Serous Otitis Media by D. Orchik, R. Morff and J. Dunn, *Archives of Otolaryngology,* 1978, *104,* 409-412. Copyright 1978 by the American Medical Association. Reprinted by permission.

ear disease in children, as well as the sensitivity, specificity, and validity of immittance audiometry in identifying middle ear disease (Jerger, 1980). Several of the above issues are beyond the scope of this chapter, while others are directly pertinent. Certainly the validity of immittance audiometry in the identification of middle ear disease is strongly supported by the previously mentioned research which involved a comparison of immittance data and findings at myringotomy (Bluestone et al., 1973; Northern & Zarnoch, 1978; Orchik, Dunn, & McNutt, 1978; Orchik, Morff, & Dunn, 1978; Renvall et al., 1980). The sensitivity of immittance to even slight changes in middle ear status is also generally accepted (Northern, 1980). Critics of immittance audiometry point to its low specificity (or high false positive rate) as its major weakness (Jerger, 1980; Northern, 1980).

The question of specificity encompasses several issues. One concerns the corroboration of the immittance findings by physical examination. Another concerns the changes in immittance data with repeated testing, either because of test-retest variability or spontaneous remission of the middle ear disease.

Immittance Audiometry and Otoscopy

When immittance testing indicates the presence of middle ear disease, the results will typically be corroborated through otoscopic examination by a physician. An important consideration is the degree of agreement one can expect between the results of immittance audiometry and otoscopy. An early investigation by McCandless and Thomas (1974) indicated excellent agreement between the two measures. Immittance data and pneumatic otoscopy were compared in 730 children, and the results of the two procedures agreed in 93% of the cases. McCandless and Thomas recommended criteria for medical referral as negative pressure in excess of -100 mmH$_2$O or an absence of the acoustic reflex. Subsequent research, however, indicated the agreement between otoscopy and immittance data was not as high as this report indicated (Konkle, Potsic, Rintelmann, Kean, & Pasquariello, 1978; Orchik, Morff, & Dunn, 1980; Roeser, Soh, Dunckel, & Adams, 1977).

Roeser et al. (1977) compared the results of otoscopy and immittance in two groups of 96 and 313 children, respectively. Children in Group I were otoscopically examined by an otologist, while children in Group II were examined by an otologist and a pediatrician. Agreement between the two procedures was much lower than previously indicated (McCandless & Thomas, 1974). Overall, the findings of the two procedures coincided in 79% of the subjects in Group I and 66% of the cases in Group II. Type C tympanograms (Jerger, 1970) accounted for the poorest agreement and, interestingly, the percentage of agreement did not improve with increasing negative pressure. Finally, interexaminer agreement for otoscopy in Group II was also poor.

The effect of physician training and prior knowledge of immittance data upon agreement between immittance audiometry and otoscopy was examined by Konkle et al. (1977). Four physicians (two otolgists and two findings and immittance data was higher than found by Roeser et al. (1977), pediatricians) were given prior instruction about immittance audiometry and interpretation of findings. Then, through a counterbalancing procedure, 73 children were examined by all four physicians. Two physicians, one from each specialty, had prior knowledge about each child's immittance data, and two did not. In general, the agreement between otoscopic indicating that prior instruction in immittance audiometry may have had an effect upon the otoscopic impressions. Prior knowledge of the immittance data also had an effect, as the percentage of ears judged abnormal by either specialist was greater when the physician had knowledge of the immittance findings prior to otoscopic examination. Finally, the percentage of ears judged abnormal increased with increasing negative pressure, also in contrast to the findings of Roeser and his associates. The number of ears judged to be otoscopically abnormal increased dramatically when negative pressure exceeded -200 mmH$_2$O.

The condition of the tympanic membrane as viewed under an operating microscope was compared to immittance data in 76 ears by Orchik et al.

(1980). The examining physician had no prior instruction in immittance audiometry, nor did he have knowledge of the immittance results. Judgments were made concerning both the plane and mobility of the tympanic membrane, and neither factor was found to be strongly related to the immittance data. The only exception was in the case of the flat or type B tympanogram (Jerger, 1970), where the condition of the tympanic membrane was judged abnormal in approximately 85% of the cases.

The preceding review suggests that the low specificity of immittance audiometry in the identification of middle ear disease is, in part, related to discrepancies between immittance data and otoscopic impressions. However, this does not necessarily constitute a weakness in immittance audiometry. As Roeser et al. (1977) have pointed out, the poor agreement is accounted for by the nature of the two procedures. Specifically, immittance audiometry is an objective measure of middle ear function, while otoscopy is a subjective measure influenced by the training and orientation of the examiner. Also, considerable deviation from normal is typically required before pathological conditions can be seen. This contention is further supported by the report of Konkle et al. (1977), which indicated that the agreement between otoscopy and immittance data was enhanced when the examining physician has had some training in immittance audiometry and has the benefit of the immittance data prior to performing the otoscopic examination. Finally, the key consideration may be what procedure is employed to define the state of the middle ear. Roeser et al. suggested changing the standard from otoscopic examination to immittance audiometry. This would allow the physician to monitor even minor changes in middle ear status that cannot be visualized through the otoscope.

Immittance Changes and Spontaneous Remission of Middle Ear Disease

Another issue involved in the question of specificity is the change in immittance findings over time. The changes in immittance data could be a result of variability in test data or spontaneous remission of the middle-ear disorder. Lewis, Dugdale, Canty, and Jerger (1975) demonstrated the day-to-day changes that can take place in tympanometric data. Ten children, aged 5 and 6 years, were tested on each of 5 consecutive days. They also examined 38 children, aged 4 to 14 years, on two occasions, 2 months apart. They found the tympanometric data changed frequently from day to day. The most variable were the Type A and Type C tympanograms using Jerger's (1970) classification. There was a 35% probability that a Type A, and a 27% probability that a Type C, tympanogram would change the following day. Type B tympanograms were much less likely to change. In the children tested 2 months apart, the greatest variability was found with negative pressure (Type C) tympanograms, as 47% of the ears showing negative pressure on initial test resolved to normal middle ear pressure at the 2-month follow-up evaluation. Lewis suggested that minor changes in middle ear pressure are to be expected, and was among the first to recommend caution in the interpretation of a single tympanogram for medical referral.

The course of Type B and C tympanograms according to Jerger's (1970) classification was examined in 3-year-old children by Fiellau-Nikolajsen and Lous (1979). A total of 504 children were screened initially. Type B or C tympanograms were found in 372 of 1,005 ears, or 37.2%. These were retested at 1 month, 3 months, and 6 months after the intial screening. The exception was that once an ear exhibited a Type A tympanogram, it was not tested further.

For Type B tympanograms, 58% remained unchanged after 1 month, with 34% remaining Type B after 3 months, while only 18% were unchanged after 6 months (Fiellau-Nikolajsen & Lous, 1979). Interestingly, Type B tympanograms were found more often and were less likely to resolve in males than females. Type C tympanograms were divided into two groups on the basis of the degree of negative pressure. Ears presenting negative pressures between -100 and -199 mmH_2O were classified as Type C_1, while Type C_2 tympanograms were those presenting negative pressures between -200 and -400 mmH_2O. Over the 6-month course, only 4% of the C_2 and 3% of the C_1 tympanograms had not changed type.

In all, 46 children showed consistently abnormal tympanograms over the 6-month course of the study (Fiellau-Nikolajsen & Lous, 1979). The children eventually underwent paracentesis, and the results were evaluated in a series of studies in terms of predictive value for otitis media, as well as prognostic value for the postoperative course (Fiellau-Nikolajsen, 1980; Fiellau-Nikolajsen, Falbe-Hansen & Knudstrup, 1980; Fiellau-Nikolajsen & Lous, 1979). Approximately 90% of the ears with preoperative Type B tympanograms were found to have significant middle ear effusion, while only 35% of ears with Type C tympanograms demonstrated this condition. Moreover, Type B tympanograms indicated the poorest prognosis, as 60% of those ears suffered a recurrence of otitis media during the 6-month postoperative period, suggesting the placement of middle ear ventilation tubes in such cases is justified.

In a separate series of studies, Tos and his colleagues (Tos, 1980; Tos, Poulsen, & Borch, 1978; Tos, Poulsen, & Hancke, 1979; Tos & Poulsen, 1980) have evaluated the spontaneous course of otitis media in children during the first 2 years of life. A number of interesting features of middle ear disorders in children were described. In general, middle ear function can be described as being quite variable during this period, beginning as normal and declining through the first year of life. The incidence of otitis media is quite high during the period from 6 months to 2 years of age, but this age period is also characterized by a high rate of spontaneous remission. Finally, the incidence of otitis media showed a definite seasonal influence, being greatest in the winter months, lower in the spring, and lowest in the summer.

The indication is, based upon the preceding research, that the low specificity of immittance audiometry in identifying middle ear disease is also related to the fluctuant status of otitis media in children. The factors producing low specificity, however, can be maintained at an acceptable level by the informed clinician. First, whenever possible, the immittance data should be combined with behavioral data. While middle ear disease does not always produce a conductive hearing loss, such a loss indicates middle ear dysfunction (Jerger & Hayes, 1980, p. 110). In cases of conductive hearing loss in children under 6 years of age, Jerger, Jerger, Mauldin, and Segal (1974) found immittance data supplemented or confirmed the conductive disorder in over 90% of the cases.

In cases where immittance data cannot be supplemented by behavioral data, the status of the middle ear should be monitored through retesting on at least one occasion several days later. This is particularly true in the application of immittance audiometry to hearing conservation programs. With the exception of children presenting Type B tympanograms (Jerger, 1970), medical referral should not be made after a single test. Further, combining tympanometry and acoustic-reflex testing should also be the screening procedure of choice.

Immittance Audiometry in the Identification of Sensorineural Hearing Loss

Jerger and Hayes (1976) have stressed the importance of employing an objective procedure as a cross-check in the use of behavioral audiometry with children. They suggested the two procedures of choice are brainstem audiometry (ABR) and immittance audiometry. In addition to its demonstrated efficiency in identifying middle ear disease in children, immittance audiometry is an important tool in the assessment of sensorineural acuity. Specifically, if one can establish the presence of normal middle ear function tympanometrically, then an estimate of sensorineural hearing level can be made using acoustic reflex threshold data.

The use of acoustic reflex data to predict hearing thresholds was first reported by Niemeyer and Sesterhenn (1974). They proposed calculating hearing thresholds using acoustic reflex thresholds for pure tones at octave frequencies from 500 through 4000 Hz, as well as for white noise. They observed that as the acoustic-reflex sensation level decreased in sensorineural hearing loss, so did the difference between the acoustic reflex threshold for pure tones and white noise.

Using the formula HL = PTAR-2.5 (PTAR-WNAR), Niemeyer and Sesterhenn (1974) contended that one could predict the average hearing level at 500 Hz through 4000 Hz (HL) by comparing the average acoustic-reflex threshold at 500 Hz through 4000 Hz (PTAR) to the acoustic-reflex threshold for white noise (WNAR). According to their data, one could predict the average pure-tone threshold at 500 Hz through 4000 Hz within ±10 dB in 73% of the cases, and within ±15 dB in 90% of the cases.

In a now classic article, Jerger and his colleagues (Jerger, Burney, Mauldin, & Crump, 1974) expanded on the work of Niemeyer and Sesterhenn in an examination of 1043 clinical patients. Jerger developed a formula based upon a comparison of the acoustic-reflex threshold for white noise and the reflex threshold for pure tones at 500, 1000, and 2000 Hz. Rather than predict average hearing levels, using Jerger's formula one could predict categories of hearing loss as shown in Table 2-2.

According to Jerger, Burney, Mauldin, and Crump (1974), the ability to predict sensorineural acuity from acoustic reflex data was related to a change in the critical bandwidth for loudness in sensorineural hearing loss as reported by Flottorp, Djupesland, and Winther (1971). The theory is based upon an assumption that the acoustic reflex threshold is loudness mediated. In the normal ear, white noise enjoys a loudness advantage which produces an acoustic reflex at significantly lower intensities. Thus, as illustrated in Figure 2-5, a widening in the critical bands for loudness, plus the loss in high frequency sensitivity usually associated with sensorineural hearing loss, would have a greater effect upon the overall loudness of white noise than for individual pure tones. The net result is a reduction in what Jerger et al. referred to as the noise-tone difference (ND). The greater the sensorineural hearing loss, the smaller the ND. The assumption of a reduced ND being related to a widening in critical band for loudness was later supported to some extent by the work of Schwartz and Sanders (1976).

Jerger's original formula was based upon the difference between the acoustic-reflex threshold for white noise and the average reflex threshold at 500 Hz through 2000 Hz, plus the absolute sound pressure level for the white noise reflex threshold (Jerger, Burney, Mauldin, & Crump, 1974). In 1043 ears, the precise category was predicted in 60% of the cases, while another 36% of the predictions were within one category. In general, when

Table 2-2
Categories of hearing loss predicted by Jerger, Burney, Mauldin, and Crump

Category	PTA at 500, 1000, and 2000 Hz[a]
Grossly Normal	< 20 dB HL
Mild-to-moderate hearing loss	20-49 dB HL
Severe hearing loss	50-85 dB HL
Profound hearing loss	>85 dB HL

[a]Categories of hearing level after Jerger, et al. 1974

NOTE: From "Predicting Hearing Loss from the Acoustic Reflex" by J. Jerger, P. Burney, L. Mauldin, & B. Crump, *Journal of Speech and Hearing Disorders,* 1974, *39,* 12-22. Copyright 1974 by the American Speech and Hearing Association. Reprinted by permission.

an error was made, it was in the direction of overpredicting the amount of hearing loss.

Predicting the slope of the audiogram by comparing acoustic reflex thresholds for noise high-pass and low-pass filtered at 2600 Hz was also proposed by Jerger, Burney, et al. (1974). However, subsequent research by Keith (1977) indicated the variability in slope prediction significantly reduced its clinical application. Keith also suggested that the use of 85 dB SPL of white noise as a reflex-eliciting signal might be an effective screening device for sensorineural hearing loss.

In 1977, Margolis and Fox published a report which compared the methods of both Niemeyer and Sesterhenn (1974) and Jerger, Burney, et al. (1974) to a third procedure developed by Popelka, Margolis, and Wiley (1976). The method is known as the bivariate plot procedure and is based upon the assumption that there are essential differences between reflex-threshold data for normal and pathological ears. The method makes use of two important relationships: the relationship between reflex threshold and stimulus bandwith, as well as the relationship between reflex threshold and the degree of hearing loss.

The bivariate plot utilizes two measures to predict hearing loss (Margolis & Fox, 1977). The reflex threshold for a pure tone is plotted on the ordinate

FIGURE 2-5
**Jerger's Theoretical Explanation for the Noise-Tone Difference in
Normal and Sensorineural Ears (From "Predicting Hearing Loss
from the Acoustic Reflex" by J. Jerger, P. Burney, L. Mauldin, and
B. Crump,** *Journal of Speech and Hearing Disorders,* **1974, 39, 12-22.
Copyright 1974 by the American Speech and Hearing Association.
Reprinted by permission.)**

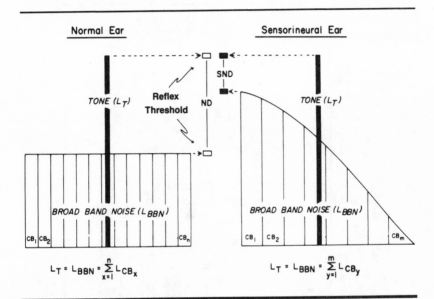

and on the abscissa is plotted the ratio between the reflex threshold for
a broad-band signal and the reflex threshold for the same pure tone. When
500 Hz and 1000 Hz pure tones were used to elicit the reflex, low-pass noise
filtered at 2600 Hz was used to arrive at the ratio. High-pass noise, also
filtered at 2600 Hz, was employed when the reflex-eliciting pure tone was
2000 Hz. Figure 2-6 illustrates the Margolis and Fox data for acoustic reflex
thresholds at 500 Hz.

The bivariate plotting procedure is more conservative than the methods
of either Niemeyer and Sesterhenn or Jerger, in that predictions are confined to either normal hearing or a "clinically significant hearing loss."
Clinically significant hearing loss was defined as a pure-tone average in
excess of 32 dB HL at 500, 1000, and 2000 Hz. According to Margolis
and Fox (1977), using the bivariate plot allowed 93% correct identification of hearing loss in excess of 32 dB. They also suggest that this procedure produces fewer false positives than the Niemeyer and Sesterhenn
and Jerger procedures.

FIGURE 2-6
Bivariate Plot of Acoustic Reflex Threshold Data at 500 Hz.
(From "Predicting Hearing Loss from the Acoustic Reflex" by
B. Margolis and M. Fox, *Journal of Speech and Hearing*
***Research,* 1977, *20,* 241-253. Copyright 1977 by the American**
Speech and Hearing Association. Reprinted by permission.)

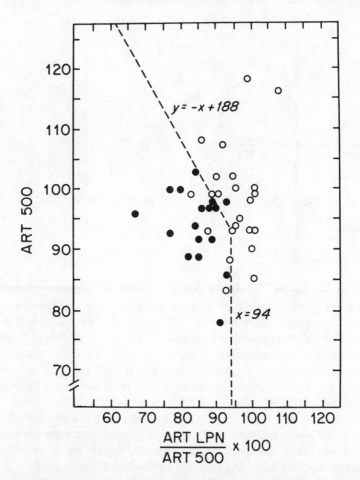

Note: The reflex threshold at 500 Hz is shown on the ordinate
in dB SPL. On the abscissa is presented 100 times the ratio
between the reflex threshold at 500 Hz. Both are expressed
in dB SPL.

Regression equations have been applied to predict hearing level from acoustic reflex data in several investigations (Baker & Lilly, 1976; Lilly, Thornton, & Baker, 1977; Rizzo & Greenberg, 1979). In each equation, reflex thresholds for broad-band noise, and as many as four pure tones, are weighted as a function of their influence upon the hearing-loss prediction. Thus, all require some mathematical manipulation of the acoustic reflex data.

The various methods of predicting hearing loss have been compared in several investigations (Hall, 1978; Hall & Koval, 1982; Keith, 1977). In general, no method is without error, although the SPAR (Sensitivity Prediction by the Acoustic Reflex) procedures developed by Jerger and his colleagues (Jerger, Burney, et al., 1974; Jerger, Hayes, & Anthony, 1978) appear to be the most popular clinical methods (Hall, 1978; Keith, 1977). This is in spite of the fact that the bivariate plotting procedure of Popelka may be somewhat more accurate in predicting hearing loss (Hall & Koval, 1982).

Regardless of which formula one employs to predict hearing level from the acoustic reflex, two important factors must be considered when utilizing acoustic reflex data with children. The factors are age and middle ear status, and each may significantly influence predictive accuracy.

Effect of Age on Predictive Accuracy

In a systematic investigation of several factors that influence the acoustic reflex, Jerger and his associates (Jerger et al., 1978) first suggested that age was a significant variable in predicting hearing loss. They observed a systematic decrease in the acoustic reflex for pure tones, but not for broad-band noise. The net effect was a gradual reduction in the noise-tone difference beyond approximately 20 years of age.

In a subsequent paper, Jerger and associates suggested that because of the interaction of age and hearing loss effects, the accuracy of his SPAR procedure was greatest in the pediatric population (Jerger, Hayes, & Anthony, 1978). In a series of 130 children between the ages of 2 and 12 years, normal hearing was predicted without error, while severe hearing loss was accurately predicted in 85% of the cases according to the criteria in Table 2-3. Mild-to-moderate hearing loss was predicted with considerably less accuracy, however, as only 54% were accurately predicted. Overall, the accuracy of prediction in children was quite impressive. As shown in Table 2-4, an error of more than one category occurred in just 1% of the cases.

While it is encouraging that the predictive accuracy of the acoustic reflex data is greatest in children, another important consideration in reviewing the effects of age concerns the developmental aspects of the acoustic reflex.

Table 2-3
Criteria for prediction of sensorineural hearing loss employed by Jerger

1000-4000 Hz Average hearing level	Criteria
0-19 dB HL	Noise-Tone difference ≥ 20 dB
	1000 Hz reflex threshold ≤ 100 dB HL
20-49 dB HL	Noise-Tone difference < 20 dB
	White-Noise reflex threshold ≤ 95 dBSPL
50-85 dB HL	Noise-Tone difference < 20 dB
	White-Noise reflex threshold ≥ 100 dBSPL

NOTE: From "Effect of Age on Prediction of Sensorineural Hearing Level from the Acoustic Reflex" by J. Jerger, D. Hayes, and L. Anthony, *Archives of Otolaryngology,* 1978, *104,* 393-394. Copyright 1978 by the American Medical Association. Reprinted by permission.

Put another way, at what age can one expect the acoustic reflex to be present in a normal-hearing child?

Abahazi and Greenberg (1977) examined the acoustic-reflex characteristics of 62 infants between the ages of 1 month and 1 year. All of the children had normal tympanograms with pressure peaks within ±50 mmH2O and were judged by a pediatrician to have otologically normal ears. In addition, all infants had been products of uncomplicated full-term pregnancies and normal deliveries. Acoustic reflex thresholds could be obtained for all stimuli (white noise, 500 Hz, 1000 Hz, 2000 Hz) in only 23 of 62 infants. Thus a prediction of hearing sensitivity could be made in only 37% of the cases. Interestingly, a slight improvement in reflex thresholds for all stimuli was also observed over the age range of 1 to 12 months. In those 23 infants for whom complete data were available, normal hearing was predicted. Thus, it would appear that in children under 1 year of age, the presence of normal acoustic reflex data would strongly suggest normal hearing, while the absence of the acoustic reflex does not necessarily imply hearing loss.

Table 2-4
Comparison of error distribution in three age groups

	AGE GROUP		
Type of Error	Children 2-12 yrs.	Young Adults 18-40 yrs.	Old Adults >59 yrs.
None, %	85	54	55
Moderate, %	14	41	41
Serious, %	1	5	4

NOTE: From "Effect of Age on Prediction of Sensorineural Hearing Level from the Acoustic Reflex" by J. Jerger, D. Hayes, and L. Anthony, *Archives of Otolaryngology,* 1978, *104,* 393-394. Copyright 1978 by the American Medical Association. Reprinted by permission.

The developmental characteristics of the acoustic reflex were also examined by Stream, Stream, Walker, and Breningstall (1978). An immittance battery was administered to 199 normal infants between birth and 15 weeks of age. In a subgroup of 90 newborn infants between 3 and 132 hours of age, the acoustic reflex could be observed in no more than 11.9% of the children. In the infants between 1 and 15 weeks of age, the occurrence of an observable acoustic reflex never exceeded 43% of the ears tested, and that represented the oldest group of infants—between 13 and 15 weeks of age.

In an examination of twenty normal infants between 18 hours and 8 days of age, Keith and Bench (1978) observed an acoustic reflex in only about 5% of the stimulus trials. A 1000 Hz pure tone, a 2600 Hz low-pass noise, and a broad-band noise were used as stimuli. In addition, reflex observance could not be facilitated by repeated signal presentation designed to habituate behavioral responses to the reflex-eliciting stimuli.

The difficulty in observing the acoustic reflex in very young children by previous researchers may have been related to probe-tone frequency rather than maturational phenomena, according to Weatherby and Bennett (1980). They examined 44 normal neonates between 10 and 169 hours of age. They employed a broad-band noise-eliciting stimulus and probe-tone frequencies between 220 and 2000 Hz. No reflexes could be observed with a 220 Hz probe tone, while a reflex was observed in all cases when probe tones from 800 Hz to 1800 Hz were employed.

Weatherby and Bennett suggested that the low impedance of the tympanic membrane at frequencies below 500 Hz shunts the high impedance of the middle ear system, obscuring the impedance change caused by the acoustic reflex. Another explanation was offered by Margolis and his colleagues (Margolis, Popelka, Handler, & Himelfarb, 1981), who suggested that the infant middle ear system is highly resistive, while the acoustic reflex using a 220 Hz probe tone is largely a result of a change in the reactive component. It would appear, then, that the failure to elicit the acoustic reflex in neonates was at least in part related to the probe tone frequency employed. Most commercial instruments employ probe tones in the vicinity of 220 Hz and, thus, are probably inappropriate for acoustic reflex determination below 3 months of age (Margolis et al., 1981).

The Effect of Middle Ear Status

The importance of normal middle ear status to predicting hearing loss from acoustic reflex data cannot be overemphasized. As Jerger has demonstrated, as little as a 5 dB air-bone gap in the probe ear can prevent the observance of an acoustic reflex (Jerger, Anthony, Mauldin, & Jerger, 1974).

Hall (1978) examined the influence of minor tympanogram abnormalities in the form of highly compliant middle ear systems upon predictive accuracy. In 36 cases presenting Type A^D tympanograms (Jerger, 1970), a sharp increase in predictive errors was noted for the SPAR.

The influence of a compliant middle ear system, as well as minimal negative pressure, was examined by Hall and Weaver (1979). In all, 212 subjects with minor tympanogram abnormalities and normal hearing were examined. Tympanogram abnormalities fell in one of four categories: highly compliant probe ear (A^D), slight negative pressure (-50 to -100 mmH2O) probe ear, bilateral compliant middle ear system (A^D), or bilateral negative pressure (-50 to -100 mmH2O).

Hall and Weaver (1979) found reflex thresholds to be elevated in all four subgroups, as shown in Figure 2-7. Although reflex thresholds were elevated for all stimuli, the effect was greatest for broad-band noise. This effect has obvious practical implications, as the net result would be a reduction in the noise-tone difference and a likely overprediction of the amount of hearing loss.

FIGURE 2-7
Effect of Minor Middle Ear Abnormalities Upon Acoustic Reflex
Thresholds for Broad-Band Noise (BBN) and Pure Tones (From
"Impedance Audiometry in a Young Population" by J. Hall and T.
Weaver, *Journal of Otolaryngology*, 1979, *8*, 3-12. Copyright 1979
by ORL Medical Publications Ltd. Reprinted by permission.)

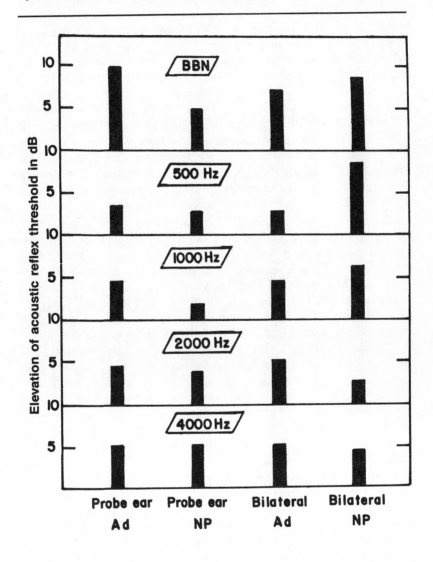

The Influence of Pressure Seal and Crossover

Two other factors that might influence predictive accuracy in children are the lack of an adequate pressure seal (Kaplan, Babecki, & Thomas, 1980; Surr & Schuckman, 1976) and acoustic reflex crossover artifact (Mahoney, 1981). Maintaining an adequate pressure seal is one of several reasons why the immittance battery cannot be completed in some children (Jerger, Jerger, Mauldin, & Segal, 1974). However, in many cases acoustic reflex data can still be obtained even without a hermetic seal.

The validity of acoustic reflex data obtained without a pressure seal was investigated by Surr and Schuchman (1976). In adults with normal hearing or sensorineural hearing loss and normal tympanograms (middle-ear pressure within ± 20 mmH$_2$O), the mean acoustic reflex thresholds with and without a pressure seal were within 2 dB for a 1000 Hz tone. In 10 children with negative middle ear pressure averaging -190 mmH$_2$O to -275 mmH$_2$O, the reflex could not be measured without a pressure seal. With a pressure seal, however, the acoustic reflex could be observed in all cases. The implication is that acoustic reflex data obtained without a pressure seal are valid only if middle ear function is normal.

Kaplan et al. (1980) examined the characteristics of the acoustic reflex with and without an hermetic seal in children with normal middle-ear function and normal hearing. Thirty children between the ages of 3 and 7 years were evaluated using as reflex-eliciting stimuli pure tones at octave intervals from 500 Hz through 4000 Hz. When present, mean acoustic reflex thresholds for sealed and unsealed conditions were not significantly different. However, in the unsealed condition, reflexes could not be observed in 33% of the ears examined at 500 and 1000 Hz, while reflexes were absent in 42% and 40% of the ears at 2000 Hz and 4000 Hz, respectively. Thus, the absence of an acoustic reflex when a pressure seal cannot be maintained is of no diagnostic value even if normal middle ear function is established. It should also be noted that Kaplan did not use a broad-band noise stimulus and, therefore, the effect of an inadequate pressure seal upon the noise-tone difference has yet to be determined. If the broad-band noise threshold is influenced differentially, then the accuracy for prediction of hearing loss could be significantly reduced.

Cross-over artifacts occur when the probe microphone picks up acoustic or vibratory energy which crosses the skull from the stimulus transducer on the contralateral side. This artifact presents as a meter deflection which is coincident with onset of the reflex-eliciting stimulus and similar to that produced by an acoustic reflex. Mahoney (1981) investigated the incidence and threshold of reflex artifact in 39 infants and children between the ages of 10 days and 6 years, 9 months. All children were fitted with earplugs which had been demonstrated in a control group to provide sufficient attenuation to eliminate the contralateral acoustic reflex. Stimuli were pure tones at octave intervals from 500 Hz to 4000 Hz, while probe-tone frequencies of 220 Hz and 660 Hz were employed.

A reflex artifact was present in every case when a 500 Hz tone was used as the eliciting stimulus with a 660 Hz probe tone. In approximately 30% of the children, a reflex artifact was present at 1000 Hz with a 660 Hz probe tone. The average artifact threshold was only 92 dB at 500 Hz and 101 dB at 1000 Hz. The reflex artifact was in evidence for the 220 Hz probe tone at 500 Hz only, where an average artifact threshold of 103 dB was found in 20% of the ears examined. It would be interesting to investigate the interaction of stimulus and probe-tone frequency using broad band noise as the stimulus, particularly in light of the report of Weatherby and Bennett (1980), who reported 100% observance of the acoustic reflex using probe tones between 800 Hz and 1800 Hz and a broad-band noise-eliciting stimulus.

Summary

Since the early reports of Brooks (1968) and Jerger (1970), immittance audiometry has received widespread application in pediatric audiology. While it is apparent that the procedure is not without error, a review of the literature suggests that with appropriate care in interpretation, immittance audiometry remains one of the most valuable tools in pediatric auditory assessment.

In the identification of middle ear disease, no measure has the sensitivity of immittance audiometry. The knowledgeable clinician, however, will remain aware of conditions of middle ear status which are subject to variability. Further, the need to combine tympanometry, acoustic reflex testing and behavioral audiometry, whenever possible, should also be emphasized. In so doing, one can take advantage of the sensitivity of immittance audiometry, while keeping the specifity at an acceptable level.

The same is true in the use of immittance audiometry in predicting sensorineural hearing level. If the clinician remains aware of the importance of establishing normal middle ear function, predictive accuracy will be enhanced. Moreover, cognizance of the age effects and the possible interaction of age and probe-tone frequency should also improve predictive accuracy.

Finally, while further research is needed in both areas of application, without doubt, immittance audiometry will continue to be an invaluable aid in the audiologic evaluation of children.

References

American National Standards Institute, Specifications for Audiometers, ANSI-S3.6 1969. New York: American National Standards Institute, 1970.

Abahazi, D.A., & Greenberg, H.J. Clinical acoustic reflex threshold measurements in infants. *Journal of Speech & Hearing Disorders.* 1977,*42*, 514-519.

Baker, S.R., & Lilly, D.J. Prediction of hearing level from acoustic reflex data. Read before the American Speech & Hearing Association Convention, Houston, November 20, 1976.

Bluestone, C., Beery, Q. & Paradise, J., Audiometry and tympanometry in relation to middle ear effusion in children. *Laryngoscope, 1973, 83,* 594-604.

Bluestone, C., Miller, M., Bess, F., et al. Panel V: Diagnosis and screening. *Annals of Otology, Rhinology & Laryngology, Suppl. 69,* 1980, *89,* 19-21.

Brooks, D. An objective method for detecting fluid in the middle ear. *International Audiology,* 1968, *7,* 280-286.

Brooks, D. Possible long-term consequences of middle ear effusion. *Annals of Otology, Rhinology and Laryngology,* Suppl. 68, 1980, *89,* 246-248.

Cantekin, E., Bluestone, C., Fria, T., Stool, S., Beery, Q. & Sabo, D. Identification of otitis media with effusion in children. *Annals of Otology, Rhinology and Laryngology,* Suppl. 68, 1980, *89,* 190-195.

Feldman, A. Tympanometry: Procedures, interpretation and variables. In A. Feldman & L. Wilber, (Eds.), *Acoustic impedance and admittance: The measurement of middle ear function.* Baltimore: Williams & Wilkins, 1976.

Fiellau-Nikolajsen, M. Serial tympanometry and middle ear status in 3-year old children. *Annals of Otology, Rhinology and Laryngology,* 1980, *42,* 220-232.

Fiellau-Nikolajsen, M., Falbe-Hansen, J., & Knudstrup, P. Tympanometry in three-year old children. *Scandinavian Audiology,* 1980, *9,* 49-54.

Fiellau-Nikolajsen, M., & Lous, J. Prospective tympanometry in three-year old children. *Archives of Otolaryngology,* 1979, *105,* 461-466.

Flottorp, G., Djupesland, G., & Winther, F. The acoustic stapedius reflex in relation to critical bandwidth. *Journal of the Acoustical Society of America,* 1971, *49,* 457-461.

Freyss, G., Narcy, P., Manac'h, Y., & Toupet, M. Acoustic reflex as a predictor of middle ear effusion. *Annals of Otology, Rhinology and Laryngology,* Suppl. 68, 1980, *89,* 196-199.

Goin, D. Acute inflammatory disease of the middle ear and mastoid. In G. English (Ed.), *Otolaryngology* New York: Harper & Row, 1975.

Hall, J.W. Predicting hearing level from the acoustic reflex. *Archives of Otolaryngology,* 1978, *104,* 601-605.

Hall, J.W., & Koval, C.B. Accuracy of hearing prediction by the acoustic reflex. *Laryngoscope,* 1982, *92,* 140-149.

Hall, J.W., & Weaver, T. Impedance audiometry in a young population. *Journal of Otolaryngology,* 1979, *8,* 3.

Holm, V., & Kunze, L. Effect of chronic otitis media on language and speech development. *Pediatrics,* 1969, *43,* 833-839.

Jerger, J. Clinical experience with impedance audiometry. *Archives of Otolaryngology,* 1970, *92,* 311-324.

Jerger, J. Dissenting report: Mass impedance screening. *Annals of Otology, Rhinology and Laryngology,* Suppl. 69, 1980, *89,* 21-22.

Jerger, J., Anthony, L., Mauldin, L., & Jerger, S. Studies in impedance audiometry: III. Middle ear disorders. *Archives of Otolaryngology,* 1974, *99,* 165-171.

Jerger, J., Burney, P., Mauldin, L., & Crump, B. Predicting hearing loss from the acoustic reflex. *Journal of Speech and Hearing Disorders,* 1974, *39,* 12-22 (1974).

Jerger, J., & Hayes, D. The crosscheck principle in pediatric audiometry. *Archives of Otolaryngology,* 1976, *102,* 614-620.

Jerger, J., & Hayes, D. Diagnostic applications of impedance audiometry: Middle ear disorder; sensorineural disorder. In J. Jerger & J. Northern (Eds.), *Clinical impedance audiometry* (2nd ed.). Acton MA: American Electromedics, 1980.

Jerger, J., Hayes, D., & Anthony, L. Effect of age on prediction of sensorineural hearing level from the acoustic reflex. *Archives of Otolaryngology,* 1978, *104,* 393-394.

Jerger, J., Hayes, D., Anthony, L., & Mauldin, L. Factors influencing prediction of hearing level from the acoustic reflex. *Monographs in Contemporary Audiology,* 1978, *1*(1).

Jerger, S., Jerger, J., Mauldin, L., & Segal, P. Studies in impedance audiometry: II. Children less than six years old. *Archives of Otolaryngology,* 1974, *99,* 1-6.

Kaplan, H., Babecki, S., & Thomas, C. The acoustic reflex in children without an hermetic seal. *Ear and Hearing,* 1980, *1,* 83-86.

Kaplan, G., Fleshman, J., Bender, T., Baum, C., & Clark, P. Long-term effects of otitis media—a ten year cohort study of Alaskan Eskimo children. *Pediatrics,* 1973, *52,* 577-585.

Keith, R. An evaluation of predicting hearing loss from the acoustic reflex. *Archives of Otolaryngology.* 1977, *103,* 419-424.

Keith, R.W., & Bench, R.J. Stapedial reflexes in neonates. *Scandanavian Audiology,* 1978, *7,* 187-191.

Konkle, D., Potsic, W., Rintelmann, W., Kean, W., & Pasquariello, P. Impedance audiometric screening in otorhinolaryngologic and pediatric practice. In E. Harford, F. Bess, C. Bluestone, & J. Klein (Eds.), *Impedance screening for middle ear disease in children.* New York: Grune & Stratton, 1978.

Lewis, N., Dugdale, A., Canty, A., & Jerger, J. Open-ended tympanometric screening: A new concept. *Archives of Otolaryngology,* 1975, *101,* 722-725.

Lilly, D.J., Thornton, A.R., & Baker, S.R. Prediction of points on the audiogram from acoustic reflex data. Paper presented at the American Speech and Hearing Association Convention, Chicago, 1977.

Mahoney, T. Acoustic reflex crossover artifacts in infants and young children. *Archives of Otolaryngology,* 1981, *107,* 363-366.

Margolis, R.H., & Fox, C.M. A comparison of three methods for predicting hearing loss from acoustic reflex thresholds. *Journal of Speech and Hearing Research,* 1977, *20,* 241-253.

Margolis, R.H., Popelka, G.R., Handler, S.D., & Himelfarb, M.Z. The effects of age on acoustic reflex thresholds in normal hearing subjects. IN G. Popelka (Ed.), *Hearing assessment with the acoustic reflex.* New York: Grune & Stratton, 1981.

McCandless, G. Impedance measures. In W.F. Rintelmann (Ed.), *Hearing assessment.* Baltimore: University Park Press, 1979.

McCandless, G., & Thomas, G. Impedance audiometry as a screening procedure for middle ear disease. *Transactions of the American Academy of Ophthalmology and Otolaryngology,* 1974, *78,* 98-102.

Metz, O. The acoustic impedance measured on normal and pathological ears. Thesis. *Acta Otolaryngologica,* Suppl. 63, 1946.

Niemeyer, W., & Sesterhenn, G. Calculating the hearing threshold from the stapedius reflex threshold for different stimuli. *Audiology,* 1974, *13,* 421-427.

Northern, J. Impedance screening: An integral part of hearing screening. *Annals of Otology, Rhinology and Laryngology,* Suppl. 68, 1980, *89,* 233-235.

Northern, J., & Downs, M. *Hearing in children* (2nd ed.). Baltimore: Williams & Wilkins, 1978.

Northern, J., & Zarnock, J. The type B tympanogram and degree of hearing loss. Paper presented at the American Speech and Hearing Association Convention, San Francisco, 1978.

Orchik, D., Dunn, J., & McNutt, L. Tympanometry as a predictor of middle ear effusion. *Archives of Otolaryngologogy,* 1978, *104,* 4-6.

Orchik, D., Morff, R., & Dunn, J. Impedance audiometry in serous otitis media. *Archives of Otolaryngology,* 1978, *104,* 409-412.

Orchik, D., Morff, R., & Dunn, J. Middle ear status at myringotomy and its relationship to the immitance battery. *Ear and Hearing,* 1980, *1,* 324-328.

Paradise, J., Smith, D., & Bluestone, C. Tympanometric detection of middle ear effusion in infants and young children. *Pediatrics,* 1976, *58,* 198-210.

Popelka, G.R., Margolis, R.H., & Wiley, T.L. Effect of activating signal bandwidth on acoustic reflex thresholds. *Journal of the Acoustical Society of America,* 1976, *59,* 153-159.

Renvall, U., Jarlstedt, J., & Holmquist, J. Identification of middle ear disease. *Acta Otolaryngology,* 1980, *90,* 283-289.

Rizzo, S., & Greenberg, H.J. Predicting hearing loss from the acoustic reflex. Read before the 50th Meeting of the Acoustical Society of America, Cambridge, MA., June 12, 1979.

Roeser, R., Soh, J., Dunckel, D., & Adams, R. Comparison of tympanometry and otoscopy in establishing pass/fail referral criteria. *Journal of the American Audiological Society,* 1977, *3,* 20-26.

Schwartz, D.M., & Sanders, J.W. Critical bandwidth and sensitivity prediction in the acoustic stapedial reflex. *Journal of Speech and Hearing Disorders,* 1976, *41,* 244-255.

Stream, R.W., Stream, K.S., Walker, J.R., & Breningstall, G. Emerging characteristics of the acoustic reflex in infants. *Otolaryngology,* 1978, *86,* 628-635.

Surr, R.K., & Schuchman, G.I. Measurement of the acoustic reflex without a pressure seal. *Archives of Otolaryngology,* 1976, *102,* 160-161.

Terkildsen, K., & Scott-Nielsen, S. An electroacoustic impedance bridge for clinical use. *Archives of Otolaryngology,* 1960, *72,* 339-

Tos, M. Spontaneous improvement of secretory otitis and impedance screening. *Archives of Otolaryngology,* 1980, *106,* 345-349.

Tos, M., & Poulsen, G. Screening tympanometry in infants and two-year old children. *Annals of Otology, Rhinology and Otolaryngology,* Suppl. 68, 1980, *89,* 217-222.

Tos, M., Poulsen, G., & Borch, J. Tympanometry in 2-year-old children. *Annals of Otology, Rhinology and Otolaryngology,* 1978, *40,* 77-85.

Tos, M., Poulsen, G., & Hancke, A. Screening tympanometry during the first year of life. *Archives of Otolaryngology,* 1979, *88,* 388-394.

Weatherby, L.A., & Bennett, M.J. The neonatal acoustic reflex. *Scandanavian Audiology,* 1980, *7,* 187-191.

Susan Jerger

Speech Audiometry

Introduction

Efforts to develop speech materials suitable for pediatric speech audiometry date back to at least the 1940s. Concurrent with the pioneering work of Carhart and Hudgins and their colleagues (summarized in Olsen & Matkin, 1979), Haskins (1949) developed word materials for speech audiometry in children. Her approach was to limit test items to words representative of the vocabulary of kindergarten children. Ten years later, in England, Watson (1957) used this same principle of test construction to generate word and sentence pediatric speech audiometric materials.

In the 1960s, Siegenthaler advanced pediatric speech-intelligibility testing by emphasizing that response paradigms, as well as test items, should be modified to conform to children's interests and abilities. He introduced the Discrimination by Identification of Pictures (DIP) test, a monosyllabic word task with a closed (picture identification) response set. Although a closed response set was employed at this time for speech threshold testing in children (spondee picture cards, toy objects), the DIP test was unique in offering a closed response set for speech discrimination testing as well.

In short, two principles, vocabulary restriction and response set definition, are important in the history of speech audiometry for children. To date, these two principles have probably been most successfully coupled in the Word Intelligibility by Picture Identification (WIPI) test of Ross and Lerman (1970).

Within the past decade, the application of diagnostic speech audiometric tests to the evaluation of central auditory disorder in adults fostered attempts to develop analogous techniques for young children (Keith, 1977). Clinical experience with pediatric central auditory testing (1) reemphasized the need to control the influence of receptive language (RL) ability on test performance and (2) highlighted the need to consider also effects of extra-auditory (cognitive) factors on children's performance. In this chapter, we detail the variety of pediatric speech audiometric procedures that have been developed within the last few years and discuss specific influences of nonauditory cognitive skills, RL ability, and chronological age on test performance.

New Test Procedures that Minimize Influence of RL Ability on Performance

Table 3-1 catalogues six new pediatric speech audiometric tests. The procedures can be divided into at least four different categories according to how they approach the problem of controlling the effect of RL ability on performance. In one approach, the influence of RL skills on behavorial audiometric results is minimized by utilizing either non-verbal signals or simplified verbal materials. Examples of this approach are the Sound Effects Recognition Test (SERT) (Finitzo-Hieber, Gerling, Matkin, & Cherow-Skalka, 1980), the Auditory Numbers Test (ANT) (Erber, 1980), and the Nonsense Syllable Discrimination Test (NSDT) (Kelley & Pillow, 1979).

In contrast to this approach, realistic speech materials are used for the remaining test procedures. However, the influence of variable RL skills on test performance is minimized in three different ways. In one approach, test materials are limited to monosyllabic words that were documented to be in the recognition vocabulary of normal children more than 2½ years old. This approach was used to develop the Northwestern University Children's Perception of Speech (Nu-chips) test (Elliott & Katz, 1980b). In the second approach, test materials represent the actual responses (internal vocabulary) of normal children between 3 and 6 years of age. The children composed both monosyllabic-word and sentence test items. Responses were elicited by picture stimulus cards selected from lists of words and actions comprising children's first vocabularies. This approach was used to develop the Pediatric Speech Intelligibility (PSI) test (Jerger, Lewis, Hawkins, & Jerger, 1980). In the third approach, test materials are based on speech samples elicited from hearing-impaired children between 8 and 15 years of age. The observed vocabulary and linguistic characteristics of the children's responses guided the construction of a battery of sentence test items. This approach resulted in the Bamford-Kowal-Bench (BKB) test (Bench & Bamford, 1979). The second column of Table 3-1 summarizes specific test materials and illustrative items for each of the procedures.

Although test materials vary widely, the testing paradigms listed in Table 3-1 (columns 3 and 4) are relatively homogeneous. With one exception, all procedures utilize a closed message set. Several previous studies (Bransford & Johnson, 1972; Kobasigawa, 1974) have documented the beneficial effect of pictorial cues on memory function. Theoretically, a closed set reduces the listener's need to store and retrieve target messages independently in memory. For five of the procedures, the message set consists of 4 to 5 alternative pictures. The child is instructed to point to the picture corresponding to the sound, word, or sentence heard. For one other test, the NSDT, target items are presented in a same-different response paradigm. The message set consists of two identical pictures that represent the "same" response mode, and two dissimilar pictures that represent the "different" response mode. The child selects one of the two alternatives. In contrast to these closed message set procedures, the BKB sentence test is routinely administered as an open message set. The child is instructed to repeat what he heard. Responses are scored as correct or incorrect on the basis of selected key words. In distinction to the routine BKB testing procedure, however, a closed message set is available for a subset of BKB test materials.

In Table 3-1, a picture identification response mode is consistently referred to as a closed message set. It should be noted, however, that pictures may not always specify target messages for young children. In particular, *abstract* picture-targets, such as fruit, may be "misread" by children as *concrete* picture-targets, e.g., apple, banana. Misreading abstract picture-targets yields a testing paradigm in which the child hears, for example, "food," and must select his or her response from the three alternatives (as the child sees them): "foot, moon, and *hamburger*." A correct response is based on the knowledge that the only alternative that represents the abstract word "food" is "hamburger." In this circumstance, a closed message set is more appropriately referred to as a closed response set. Closed message sets and closed response sets are not distinguished in this chapter.

In the fourth column of Table 3-1, the term "task domain" (TD) refers to the "gestalt" of the message set. A TD is considered *restricted* when (1) each target item is specified for the listener and (2) foil items are not included. An example of a current adult audiologic test utilizing a restricted TD is the Synthetic Sentence Identification (SSI) procedure (Speaks & Jerger, 1965). In contrast, a TD is considered *unrestricted* when target items are not uniquely specified for the listener, but are embedded among selected foil items. In this circumstance, the TD is defined, but not restricted. An

Table 3-1.
Selected Pediatric Speech Audiometric Procedures

Test	Materials	Message Set: Response Mode	Task Domain	Minimum Age (yrs.)
SERT[a]	30 Environmental sounds, (train, telephone)	*Closed:* Picture identification	*Unrestricted:* 4 alternatives	3
ANT[b]	Numbers 1 through 5	*Closed:* Picture identification	*Restricted:* 5 alternatives	3
NSDT[c]	50 Syllable pairs, (ma-la, la-la)	*Closed:* Same-Different	*Restricted:* 2 alternatives	4½
NU-CHIPS[d]	50 Mono-syllabic words, (nose, school)	*Closed:* Picture identification	*Unrestricted:* 4 alternatives	3
PSI[e]	20 Mono-syllabic words, (dog, spoon)	*Closed:* Picture identification	*Restricted:* 5 alternatives	3

| PSIe | 10 Sentences, 2 syntactic constructions (Show me a bear brushing his teeth.) (A bear is brushing his teeth.) | Closed: Picture identification | Restricted: 5 alternatives | 3 |
| BKBf | 336 Sentences, (A cat sits on the bed.) | Open: Verbal repetition | Unspecified: Unknown alternatives | 8 |

NOTE: For a definition of each test's acronym, see text.

aFinitzo-Hieber, Gerling, Matkin, & Cherow-Skalka, 1980.

bErber, 1980.

cKelley & Pillow, 1979.

dElliott & Katz, 1980b.

eJerger, Lewis, Hawkins, & Jerger, 1980.

fBench & Bamford, 1979.

example of a current pediatric audiologic test with an unrestricted TD is the Word Intelligibility by Picture Identification (WIPI) procedure (Ross and Lerman, 1970). Finally, a TD is considered *unspecified* when possible targets are not defined for the listener. An example of an unspecified TD is the traditional adult monosyllabic (PB) word test. Both restricted and unrestricted TDs are closed message set procedures, whereas an unspecified TD is an open message set procedure. Of the procedures listed in Table 3-1, four involve restricted TDs, two involve unrestricted TDs, and one is an unspecified TD. The Sert and Nu-chips tests are described as unrestricted TDs because each target is embedded in a different message set of selected foil items. However, it should be noted that both of these tests interchange target and foil items. For example, the Nu-chips test consists of 65 word pictures: 50 words are used interchangably as targets and foils, and 15 words are foils only. The advantages and disadvantages of restricted versus unrestricted TDs are discussed later in this chapter.

The last column in Table 3-1 specifies the minimum age for administering the test procedures. With two exceptions, the newly developed procedures are appropriate for children as young as 3 years of age. The exceptions are the NSDT test, which is limited to children above 4½ years old, and the BKB sentence test, which is designated for children at least 8 years of age.

In short, a variety of test procedures is presently available for pediatric audiometric evaluations. The procedures represent at least four different approaches to minimizing the effect of RL ability on speech intelligibility performance.

Next, we examine the possible influence of developing cognitive skills and chronological age on results of behavioral speech audiometry.

Effect of Nonauditory Abilities

In addition to auditory factors, certain nonauditory cognitive factors may affect performance on pediatric speech audiometric procedures. Several of the investigators listed in Table 3-1 attempted to minimize the effect of nonauditory factors on test performance. A test condition that appears to have received primary emphasis in these studies is the TD.

Advantages and Disadvantages of Restricted vs. Unrestricted TDs

The advantages of a restricted TD primarily concern the conceptual processing of speech signals. More specifically, a listener's interpretation of speech signals is based on two different, interactive processing strategies:(1) a physical (*bottom-up*) analysis, triggered by the arrival of sensory information, and (2) a conceptual (*top-down*) processing mechanism, triggered by the person's general knowledge and expectations based on the context of the sensory event (Marslen-Wilson & Welsh, 1978; Norman, 1976). Theoretically, a restricted closed message set aids the conceptual *top-down* processing of speech messages. A restricted TD specifies for the listener what he may expect to hear.

A restricted TD also aids the attentional-memory factors required in speech tasks. For example, with a restricted TD, a child can name and briefly elaborate each target item before testing begins. Theoretically, active verbal processing assists (1) in encoding all target messages at a more constant depth of processing, and (2) in neutralizing differences in perceptual salience. Consider an illustrative test condition with four alternative items: "dog, pig, wolf, and cat." Initially, before verbal elaboration, a young child with a favorite dog in her home may attend to and identify the word and picture of "dog" more readily than the other alternatives. The representation of the dog has *increased perceptual salience* for her. However, if the child elaborates each target picture with her parent or a clinician before testing (i.e., briefly discusses the three little *pigs*, the big bad *wolf*, etc.), the effect of perceptual salience on performance is theoretically minimized. The effectiveness of verbal labeling and elaboration as an attentional-mnemonic device has been discussed by several investigators (Luszcz and Bacharach, 1980; Miller & Johnson-Laird, 1976; Norman, 1976).

In contrast to a restricted TD, each target in an unrestricted TD is embedded in a different closed message set. A large number of alternative items are typically involved. A disadvantage of an unrestricted TD is that it is impractical to label and elaborate each possible item verbally. Consequently, active verbal processing cannot be used to minimize the effects of attentional-memory factors on test performance. A further complication is that young children may verbally label and elaborate an item (picture) with increased perceptual salience spontaneously. For example, when a page is turned to a new item and new closed message set, young children frequently point to one picture and say it aloud ("gun, bang, bang"). In this circumstance, differences in depth of processing and perceptual salience may affect test results in some children.

This viewpoint is supported by data relating performance on behavioral tests sensitive to prefrontal cortex function in children and in adults or animals with lesions. Rose (1980) recently reviewed the literature in this area. Results show that children below about 5 years of age perform like lesioned animals or adults on behavioral tests involving prefrontal cortex function. A primary finding is that humans or animals with dysfunction or immaturity of the prefrontal cortex are unable to inhibit their initial response tendency during a task. This finding is consistent with Luria's (1973) observation that the prefrontal cortex in humans begins to mature at about 5 to 7 years of age.

These results are important to the clinical evaluation of speech intelligibility performance in children for primarily one reason. If children with prefrontal cortex immaturity are unable to inhibit their first available response during a task, then performance on a test with an unrestricted TD may unduly reflect a child's initial response tendency (e.g., to attend and respond preferentially to "dog"), *rather than what he or she heard.* Clinicians who have administered tests with unrestricted TDs (e.g., the WIPI test) may recall older children who initially point to one picture and then change their response to another alternative. Maturation of prefrontal cortex function may be allowing the child to alter, although not yet inhibit, his or her first available response. However, younger children, less than about 5 years of age, may not be able to alter an initial response tendency during a task. Relative to performance in a restricted TD, performance in an unrestricted TD may be more influenced by effects of perceptual salience in some children.[1]

In spite of the above observations, some clinicians criticize restricted TD procedures, noting that restricted targets may not require the child to discriminate phonetic/acoustic information. For example, in the previous illustrative restricted TD ("dog, pig, wolf, and cat"), a child may theoretically discriminate among the response alternatives on the basis of either an isolated consonant or vowel segment. Toward this criticism, some clinicians select unrestricted TDs. An unrestricted condition allows one to embed target items in carefully constructed foil items that represent selected phonemic confusions. For example, the target item "cat" may be embedded among foil items of "hat, fat, and rat." It should be noted, however, that the degree of contrast and the position of contrastive phonemes characterizing foil items may influence task difficulty for children. Interested readers are referred to Lenel and Cantor (1981).

In short, investigators oriented toward the conceptual processing of speech signals may prefer restricted TDs with a limited number of target items. Other investigators, however, oriented toward the phonological processing of speech signals may prefer unrestricted TDs with foil items. One exception to the above two philosophical distinctions may involve the new NSDT test (Table 3-1). This procedure with a same-different response paradigm may represent an alternative approach that allows clinicians to study phonological aspects of speech understanding without the disadvantages of an unrestricted (foil-item) TD.

Effect of Maturation

Developmental changes in speech intelligibility performance have been well documented for at least 13 years. Age-related improvements in performance have been reported for degraded nonsense syllables (Nagafuchi, 1976), unaltered or degraded word materials[2] and unaltered or degraded sentence materials[3]. Additionally, age-related changes have been observed in studies of the acoustic-phonetic cues underlying speech perception. Increasing performance with increasing age has been reported for format frequency difference limens (Eguchi, 1976), for voice onset time (Eilers, Wilson, & Moore, 1979), and for detection and identification thresholds of synthesized consonant vowel (CV) syllables (Elliott, Longinotti, Meyer, Raz, & Zucker, 1981).

Previous investigators have emphasized that the observed developmental changes in speech understanding ability may be associated with the maturation of many different auditory and nonauditory skills. Increasing performance with increasing age has been related to growth in (1) basic cognitive skills and the ability to adopt more appropriate task-processing strategies[4], (2) specific language processing skills[5], (3) the amount and organization of information in the child's knowledge base and his or her overall information-processing capacity (Berlin, Hughes, Lowe-Bell, & Berlin, 1973; Keating, Keniston, Manis, & Bobbitt, 1980), (4) the ability to attend selectively to relevant information[6], (5) the discrimination of acoustic cues and the linguistic organization of acoustic patterns[7], and (6) auditory sensitivity[8]. Theoretically, the above components of the maturational process may render the speech perception mechanism more resistant to degradation in relatively older individuals.

Table 3-2 illustrates the degree of maturational change that characterizes speech intelligibility performance in children less than 7 years old. Results for PSI speech materials were selected for this illustrative example. Table 3-2 details average performance for PSI sentence and word materials as a function of chronological age. Subjects were normal children between 3 and 6 years of age. For these data, sentence and word items were presented at 50 dB sound pressure level (SPL). The listening task was made difficult by measuring performance in the presence of a competing speech message. The message-to-competition ratio (MCR) was 0 dB for sentence materials and +4 dB and 0 dB for word materials. For the latter condition, performance was averaged across the two MCR conditions because results at +4 dB MCR were 95-100% in all age groups. Consequently, any age effects could not be observed at this MCR. The absolute percent-correct scores averaged across +4 and 0 dB MCRs approximated the absolute correct levels for sentence results.

Table 3-2.
Average Performance for PSI Sentence and Word Materials as a
Function of Chronological Age

Chronological age (years)	Sentences (%) (Format II)	Sentences (%) (Varied Format)	Monosyllabic Words (%)
6-0 to 6-11	94	94	87
5-0 to 5-11	89	94	81
4-0 to 4-11	83	89	78
3-0 to 3-11	63	79	75
Difference	31	15	12

NOTE: Test items were presented at 50 dB sound pressure level. For sentences, data represent results at a message-to-competition ratio (MRC) of 0 dB. For words, data are average results at MCRs of +4 dB and 0 dB. Subjects were normal children between 3 and 6 years of age (N=42 for sentences and N=40 for words).

In Table 3-2, sentence results are presented for a constant format (Format II) and varied format (Format I or Format II) materials (see Table 3-1 for illustrative examples). For the varied sentence format condition, the appropriate test materials were selected according to the child's RL ability. Children with relatively low RL skill were tested with Format I sentences; children with relatively high RL ability were tested with Format II sentences. The purpose of varying the sentence format as a function of the child's RL skills is to minimize the influence of RL ability on performance. (Please see Jerger, Jerger, & Lewis, 1981, for further detail.) For word results, all children were tested with the same monosyllabic word items. RL ability does not appear to affect performance for PSI word materials (Jerger et al., 1981).

As seen in Table 3-2, average performance for Format II sentences improved 31% as age increased from 3 to 6 years. Average performance was 94% in the 6-year-olds, but only 63% in the 3-year-olds. However, when the sentence format was varied according to the child's RL ability, performance improved only 15% as age increased from 3 to 6 years. Average performance for adjusted-format sentences was 94% in the 6-year-olds and 79% in the 3-year-olds. In other words, varying the sentence format as a function of the child's RL ability reduced the previously observed performance difference for Format II sentences by about one-half, from 31%

to 15%. Average performance for PSI word materials increased 12% with increasing age. Average scores were 87% in the 6-year-olds and 75% in the 3-year-olds. Notice that the degree of maturational change was similar for word materials and adjusted-format sentence materials. The degree of maturational change characterizing PSI speech materials is similar to results of previous developmental studies (Palva & Jokinen, 1975, Schwartz & Goldman, 1974; Siegenthaler, 1969).

In the following section, we examine pediatric speech audiometric procedures from a psychophysical viewpoint. For this review, we detail characteristics of normal performance-intensity (PI) functions for different pediatric speech materials. Several of the procedures shown in Table 3-1 are not included in this review, because normative PI functions for the test materials are not available.

Psychophysical Data

Performance-Intensity (PI) Functions for Monosyllabic Words

Table 3-3 tabulates the steepness and threshold characteristics of PI functions for six pediatric monosyllabic word tests. Selected procedures are the PB-Kindergarten (PB-K) test (Haskins, 1949), the AB test (Boothroyd, 1968), the DIP test (Siegenthaler, 1969), the Gottinger test (Chilla et al., 1976), the Nu-chips test (Elliott & Katz, 1980b), and the PSI test (Jerger et al., 1980). Subjects were normal children between 3 and 6 years of age. For five tests, data are grouped according to chronological age. For the PSI test, however, results are grouped according to RL ability (even though all children were tested with the same word materials). The Receptive Language Level I (RLL I) group consists of children with scores on the Northwestern Syntax Screening Test (NSST) of less than 32; the RLL II group is composed of children with NSST scores of greater than or equal to 32. Note that the PSI test is routinely administered in isolation and in the presence of a competing speech message. For comparative purposes, normal data for adult monosyllabic word materials are presented.

Table 3-3a summarizes steepness characteristics for the six pediatric speech intelligibility procedures. Table entries represent the intensity range in dB corresponding to the performance range from 20% to 80%. Data were obtained by plotting PI functions on normal probability paper and visually determining a best-fit linear function. Steepness characteristics are summarized by the dB range yielding 20% to 80%, rather than the conventional percentage-per-dB approach, because we did not want steepness estimates from other investigators to be subjected to an additional transformation.

Table 3-3.
Steepness and Threshold Characteristics of Performance-Intensity Functions for Six Pediatric Monosyllabic Word Tests

Subjects were normal children between 3 and 6 years of age. For five tests, data are grouped according to chronological age (3-4 years and 5-6 years). For the PSI test, however, results are grouped according to receptive language level (RLL I and RLL II). The RLL I group consists of children with NSST scores of less than 32; the RLL II group consists of children with NSST scores of greater than or equal to 32. Notice that the PSI is administered in isolation and in the presence of a competing speech message (CM). For comparative purposes, normal data for adult monosyllabic word materials are presented.

Table 3-3a.
Steepness Characteristics

Word Materials	Groups	
	(3 - 4-year-olds)	*(5 - 6-year-olds)*
PB-K Test[a]	--	14
A.B. Test[b]	--	15
DIP Test[c]	14	12
Gottinger Test[d]	14	10
Nu-Chips Test[e]	21	18
	(RLL I)	*(RLL II)*
PSI[f]	10	8
PSI:CM[f]	12	10
Adult Words[g]	11 - 15	

NOTE: Table entries represent the intensity range in dB corresponding to the performance range from 20 to 80%.

[a]Personal unpublished data, 1980.

[b]Boothroyd, 1968.

[c]Siegenthaler, 1969. Data obtained by plotting author's results from about 40-80% on normal probability paper and extrapolating down to 20%.

[d]Chilla et al., 1976.
[e]Elliott & Katz, 1980b. Data obtained by plotting author's results from about 50-80% on normal probability paper and extrapolating down to 20%.
[f]Jerger & Jerger, 1982.
[g]Olsen & Matkin, 1979.

For five of the six procedures in Table 3-3a, the performance range defining 20% to 80% correct was 8-15 dB. The exception involves the Nu-chips word materials. The steepness of PI functions for the Nu-chips materials appears to be more gradual than the steepness of other pediatric word tests. For the Nu-chips test, the performance range between 20% and 80% is 21 dB in 3-year-olds and 18 dB in 5-year-olds. In general, for all procedures, PI-word functions are about 2-4 dB steeper in older children than in younger children. In adults, the intensity range corresponding to 20-80% correct for monosyllabic word materials ranges from about 11 to 15 dB (Olsen & Matkin, 1979). Relative to the steepness of adult word materials, the steepness of pediatric PI functions is slightly increased for the PSI test; is comparable for the Gottinger test, the AB test, the DIP test, and the PB-K test; and is flatter for the Nu-chips test. Differences in the steepness of PI functions may be due to a variety of auditory and nonauditory factors, such as differences in the (1) influence of cognitive skills on the task, (2) homogeneity of test items, (3) scoring techniques (e.g., words vs. phonemes), (4) perceptual salience of the verbal materials, (5) number of test items per trial, etc. Some of these factors have been discussed previously by Bench and Bamford and their colleagues (Bench & Bamford, 1979).

Table 3-3b shows the threshold values, or 50% correct level, in dB SPL, for the six pediatric monosyllabic word procedures. Again, with the exception of the PSI test, results are grouped according to chronological age. For the PSI test, data are grouped according to RL level. For comparative purposes, data for adult word materials are presented. With two exceptions, speech thresholds for the pediatric word tests range from 18 dB to 29 dB SPL. The exceptions are the unusually sensitive threshold, 14 dB SPL, observed for Threshold by Identification of Pictures (TIP) monosyllabic words in 5 to 6-year-olds and the unusually poor speech threshold, 37 dB SPL, observed for PB-K words in the same age group. A difference of about 20 dB between PB-K speech thresholds and other speech thresholds suggests that the PB-K word test is a more difficult listening task for children. However, as shown in Table 3-3a, the steepness of the PI function for PB-K words was not unusually flat relative to other pediatric monosyllabic word materials. Bench and Bamford (1979)

Table 3-3b
Threshold Values (50% Correct Level) in Sound Pressure Level (dB SPL)

Word Materials	Groups	
	(3 - 4-year-olds)	*(5 - 6-year-olds)*
PB-K Test[a]	--	37
A.B. Test[b]	--	20
TIP Test[c]	18	14
Gottinger Test[d]	26	20
Nu-Chips Test[e]	29	24
	(RLL I)	*(RLL II)*
PSI[f]	23	22
PSI:CM[f]	26	25
Adult Words[g]	24-31	

[a] Personal unpublished data, 1980
[b] Boothroyd, 1968.
[c] Siegenthaler, 1969.
[d] Chilla et al., 1976.
[e] Elliott & Katz, 1980b. Data obtained by converting sensation level results to hearing level (HL) by adding mean SRT for group, then converting HL to SPL (0 dB HL = 20 dB SPL).
[f] Jerger & Jerger, 1982.
[g] For references, see text.

suggest that a threshold difference without a steepness difference does not indicate a more difficult speech task, but simply indicates a calibration error. However, the PB-K threshold reported in Table 3-3b is consistent with extrapolated results for previous PB-K threshold estimations in 5 to 6-year-old children (Beasley, Maki, & Orchik, 1976; Elliott & Katz, 1980b). With the exception of PB-K and TIP results, the speech thresholds reported in Table 3-3b are in general agreement with the speech thresholds observed for monosyllabic word materials in adults, about 24 to 31 dB SPL (Hirsh et al., 1952; Jerger & Jerger, 1976; Niemeyer, 1965; Speaks, 1967).

Performance-Intensity (PI) Functions for Sentences

With the exception of the PSI test, pediatric sentence procedures are not available for children less than about 8-10 years old. For this reason, in this section, the PSI sentence test is necessarily compared to older child-adult sentence materials. This limitation suggests, however, that further research on sentence intelligibility tests in young children is needed.

Table 3-4 tabulates the steepness and threshold characteristics of PI functions for five sentence tests—the Manchester test (Watson, 1957), Fry test (Fry, 1961), Synthetic Sentence Identification (SSI) test (Speaks & Jerger, 1965), BKB picture-related test (Bench & Bamford, 1979), and PSI test (Jerger et al., 1980). For four tests, subjects were normal children between 10 and 15 years of age. For the PSI test, however, subjects were normal children between 3 and 6 years. For the latter test, subjects are grouped according to receptive language level (RLL). The RLL I group was tested with Format I sentences; the RLL II group was tested with Format II sentences. Note that the PSI test is routinely administered in isolation and in the presence of a competing speech message. For comparative purposes, normal data for sentence materials in adults are presented.

Table 3-4a summarizes steepness characteristics for the five tests. Table entries are the intensity range in dB corresponding to the performance range yielding 20 - 80% correct. Data were determined from the line of best fit for PI functions as plotted on probability paper. The performance range defining 20-80% was 8-11 dB for PSI sentence materials, 12-13 dB for the Fry and Manchester sentence materials, and 15-17 dB for the BKB-picture test and the SSI materials in the presence of a competing message at 0 dB MCR. One comment concerning the BKB-picture test is that subsequent testing in children with hearing loss (Bench, Bamford, Wilson, & Clifft, 1979) yielded a steeper function, about 13 dB. If one assumes that the PI function in normal listeners should theoretically be steeper, or at least as steep as PI functions in children with hearing loss, then the normal data of Bamford and Wilson (1979) reported in Table 3-4a may be somewhat spurious.

In adults, the intensity range yielding 20%-80% is 5-7 dB for SSI sentences in isolation, first order approximations (Speaks, 1967; Speaks, Jerger & Jerger, 1966) and third-order approximations (Jerger, 1980; Speaks, Karmen, & Benitez, 1967); 7 dB for German sentences in quiet (Niemeyer, 1965); and 19 dB for SSI materials (third-order approximations) in competition (0 dB MCR) (Jerger, 1980). With regard to PI functions in isolation, results for pediatric PI functions are more gradual than results for adult sentence materials. In contrast, PI functions for PSI sentence materials in competition are relatively steeper. The steepness of SSI functions (0 dB MCR) in older children versus adults is comparable.

Table 3-4
Steepness and Threshold Characteristics of Performance-Intensity Functions for Five Sentence Tests

> For four tests, subjects were normal children between 10 and 15 years of age. For the PSI test, subjects were normal children between 3 and 6 years of age. For the latter test, subjects are grouped according to receptive language level (RLL). The RLL I group (NSST scores of less than 32) was tested with Format I sentences; the RLL II group (NSST scores of greater than or equal to 32) was tested with Format II sentences. Note that the SSI test is routinely administered in the presence of a competing message (CM) and that the PSI test is routinely administered in isolation and in competition (CM). For comparative purposes, normal data for adult sentence materials are included.

Table 3-4a
Steepness Characteristics

Sentence Materials	Groups	
	---	(10 - 15-year-olds)
Fry Test[a]	---	12
Manchester Test[a]	---	13
BKB-Picture Test[a]	---	15
SSI:CM[b]	---	17
	(RLL I)	(RLL II)
PSI$_c$	8	9
PSI:CM[c]	10	11
Adult Sentences[d]		5-7
Adult Sentences: CM[b]		19

NOTE: Table entries represent the intensity range in dB corresponding to the performance range from 20 to 80%.

[a]Bamford and Wilson, 1979.

bPersonal unpublished data, 1980.

cJerger & Jerger, 1982.

dFor references, see text.

Table 3-4b
Threshold Values (50% Correct Level) in Sound Pressure Level (dB SPL)

Sentence Materials	Groups	
	---	(10 - 15-year-olds)
Fry Test[a]	---	31
Manchester Test[a]	---	32
BKB-Picture Test[a]	---	30
SSI:CM[b]	---	34
	(RLL I)	*(RLL II)*
PSI[c]	21	21
PSI:CM[c]	26	21
Adult Sentences[d]		16-18
Adult Sentences: CM[b]		31

aBamford & Wilson, 1979.

bPersonal unpublished data, 1980.

cJerger & Jerger, 1982.

dFor references, see text.

Table 3-4b shows speech thresholds, or the 50% correct level, in dB SPL, for the five sentence tests. With one exception, thresholds for the sentence materials ranged from 30 to 34 dB SPL. The exception concerns the more sensitive speech thresholds observed for PSI sentence materials. The PSI sentence thresholds in isolation and in the presence of a competing message ranged from 21 to 26 dB SPL in both subject groups. In adults, thresholds are about 16-18 dB SPL for sentences in isolation (Jerger, 1980; Niemeyer, 1965; Speaks, 1967) and 31 dB SPL for SSI sentences (third-order approximations) in competition (0 dB MCR) (Jerger, 1980).

In Tables 3-3 and 3-4, performance for PSI word versus sentence materials may be contrasted. Comparison of the steepness of PSI word versus sentence functions within each subject group (Tables 3-3a and 3-4a) reveals that steepness characteristics were statistically equivalent (p.>.05) in isolation and in competition. This finding is not consistent with previous results on adult speech materials (summarized at bottom of tables 3-3a and 3-4a). In adults, PI functions for sentences are characteristically steeper than PI functions for words.

In general correspondence with steepness results, threshold values for PSI words versus sentences (Tables 3-3b and 3-4b) were also statistically equivalent (p>.05) within each subject group, with the exception of the competing condition in the RLL II group. In the RLL II group, a more sensitive threshold value was observed for sentences than for words in the presence of competing speech. Only this latter finding is consistent with previous results obtained with word and sentence materials in adults (summarized at the bottom of Tables 3-3b and 3-4b).

In relating performance for words versus sentences on the PSI test to previous findings in adults, it should be remembered that word and sentence performance in adults has traditionally been studied with one or both of the speech materials presented in an open, rather than a closed, message set. Consequently, results based on adult speech materials may not be applicable to PSI results in children. This viewpoint is supported by Wilson and Antablin's (1980) demonstration that a closed message set paradigm noticeably increased the steepness and improved the threshold of monosyllabic word PI functions in adults.

In overview, normative data for speech intelligibility tests in children indicate that the steepness of PI functions, defined by the intensity range yielding performance between 20% and 80%, ranges from 8 to 21 dB for word items and from 8 to 17 dB for sentence materials. Threshold values, 50% correct level, range from 14 to 37 dB SPL for word materials and from 21 to 34 dB SPL for sentence messages.

Summary

1. Recent advances in pediatric speech intelligibility procedures have yielded a wide variety of available tests representing at least four different approaches to minimizing the effect of receptive language ability on speech audiometric performance.

2. Current pediatric speech audiometric procedures are presented in either unspecified, unrestricted, or restricted task domains. An unrestricted task domain may be preferred by individuals oriented toward phonological aspects of speech processing; a restricted task domain may be preferred by individuals oriented toward conceptual aspects of speech processing. Both unrestricted and restricted task domains have advantages and disadvantages that clinicians must consider in individual testing conditions.

3. Receptive language ability, cognitive skills, and chronological age may effect performance on pediatric speech intelligibility tests.

4. For six pediatric monosyllabic word tests in normal children between 3 and 6 years, the steepness of PI functions, defined by the intensity range yielding performance between 20% and 80%, ranged from 8 to 21 dB. Threshold values, 50% correct level, ranged from 14 to 37 dB SPL.

5. For five sentence tests in normal children between 3 and 15 years old, the steepness of PI functions ranged from 8 to 17 dB and threshold values ranged from 21 to 34 dB SPL.

Notes

[1]Recently, I was administering a picture identification speech test with an unrestricted TD to a 3-year-old. Often, when the page was turned to a new messsage set, she would verbally label and elaborate one item. We couldn't get her to stop. Finally, I said to her 5-year-old sister, "Why does she keep talking?" Her sister replied, "She's not talking, she's reading. Mommy likes her to do that at home. If you don't want her to read, don't give her a book."

[2]Beasley et al., 1976; Elliott & Katz, 1980; Fior, 1972; Goldman et al., 1970; Jerger et al., 1981; Palva & Jokinen, 1975; Sanderson-Leepa & Rintelmann, 1976; Schwartz & Goldman, 1974; Siegenthaler, 1969; Siegenthaler, 1975; Smith & Hodgson, 1970; Willeford, 1977.

[3]Beasley & Flaherty-Rintelmann, 1976; Costello, 1977; Entwisle & Frasure, 1974; Jerger et al., 1981; Marshall et al., 1979; Nelson, 1976; Schwartz & Goldman, 1974; Teatini, 1970; Willeford, 1981.

[4]Hagen, 1972; Halford & Wilson, 1980; Keating et al., 1980; Kramer et al., 1980.

[5]Entwisle & Frasure, 1974; Frasure & Entwisle, 1973; Marshall et al., 1979; Nelson, 1976.

[6]Anooshian & Prilop, 1980; Doyle, 1973; Geffen & Sexton, 1978; Zukier & Hagen, 1978.

[7]Boothroyd, 1970; Carpenter, 1976; Simon & Fourcin, 1978.

[8]Elliott & Katz, 1980a; Fior, 1972; Jerger et al., 1981; Palva & Jokinen, 1975; Siegenthaler, 1969.

Acknowledgments

Preparation of this chapter was supported by Public Health Service Clinical Research Center grant NS-10940 from the National Institute of Neurological and Communicative Disorders and Stroke. I thank my friends at Arizona State University, Dr. Maureen Hannley and Dr. Michael Dorman, and at Baylor College of Medicine for their critical review of the initial version of this chapter.

References

Anooshian, L., & Prilop, L. Developmental trends for auditory selective attention: dependence on central-incidental word relations. *Child Development*, 1980, *51*, 45-54.

Bamford, J., & Wilson, I. Methodological considerations and practical aspects of the BKB sentence lists. In J. Bench & J. Bamford (Eds.), *Speech-hearing tests and the spoken language of hearing-impaired children*. London: Academic Press, 1979, 147-187.

Beasley, D., & Flaherty-Rintelmann, A. Children's perception of temporally distorted sentential approximations of varying length, *Audiology*, 1976, *15*, 315-325.

Beasley, D., Maki, J., & Orchik, D. Children's perception of time-compressed speech on two measures of speech discrimination. *Journal of Speech and Hearing Disorders*, 1976, *41*, 216-225.

Bench J., & Bamford, J. *Speech-hearing tests and the spoken language of hearing-impaired children*. London: Academic Press, 1979.

Bench, J., Bamford, J., Wilson, I., & Clifft, L. A comparison of the BKB sentence lists for children with other speech audiometry tests. *Australian Journal of Audiology*, 1979, *1*, 61-66.

Berlin, C., Hughes, L., Lowe-Bell, S., & Berlin, H. Dichotic right ear advantage in children 5 to 13. *Cortex*, 1973, *9*, 393-401.

Boothroyd, A. Developments in speech audiometry. *Sound*, 1968, *2*, 3-11.

Boothroyd, A. Developmental factors in speech recognition. *Audiology*, 1970, *9*, 30-38.

Bransford, J., & Johnson, M. Contextual prerequisites for understanding: Some investigations of comprehension and recall. *Journal of Verbal Learning Behavior*, 1972, *11*, 717-726.

Carpenter, R. Development of acoustic cue discrimination in children. *Journal of Communication Disorders*, 1976, *9*, 7-17.

Chilla, R., Gabriel, P., Kozielski, P., Bansch, D., & Kabas, M. Der Gottinger Kindersprachverstandnistest. I. Sprachaudiometrie des "kindergarten"—Und retardierten Kindes mit einem Einsilber-Bildtest. *H.N.O.*, 1976, *24*, 342-346.

Costello, M. Evaluation of auditory behavior of children using the Flowers-Costello test of central auditory abilities. In R. Keith (Ed.), *Central auditory dysfunction*, New York: Grune & Stratton, 1977, 257-276.

Doyle, A. Listening to distraction: A developmental study of selective attention. *Journal of Experimental Child Psychology*, 1973, *15*, 100-115.

Eguchi, S. Difference limens for the formant frequencies: Normal adult values and their development in children. *Journal of American Auditory Society*, 1976, *1*, 145-149.

Eilers, R., Wilson, W., & Moore, J. Speech discrimination in the language-innocent and the language-wise: A study in the perception of voice onset time. *Journal of Child Language*, 1979, *6*, 1-18.

Elliott, L., & Katz, D. Children's pure-tone detection, *Journal of the Acoustical Society of America*, 1980, *67*, 343-344. (a)

Elliott, L., & Katz, D. *Development of a new children's test of speech discrimination*. St. Louis: Auditec, 1980. (b)

Elliott, L., Longinotti, C., Meyer, D., Raz, I., & Zucker, K. Developmental differences in identifying and discriminating CV syllables. *Journal of the Acoustical Society of America*, 1981, *70*, 669-677.

Entwisle, D., & Frasure, N. A contradiction resolved: Children's processing of syntactic cues. *Developmental Psychology,* 1974, *10,* 852-857.

Erber, N. Use of the auditory numbers test to evaluate speech perception abilities of hearing-impaired children. *Journal of Speech and Hearing Disorders,* 1980, *45,* 527-532.

Finitzo-Hieber, T., Gerling, I., Matkin, N., & Cherow-Skalka, E. A sound effects recognition test for the pediatric audiological evaluation. *Ear and Hearing,* 1980, *1,* 271-276.

Fior, R. Physiological maturation of auditory function between 3 and 13 years of age. *Audiology,* 1972, *11,* 317-321.

Frasure, N., & Entwisle, D. Semantic and syntactic development in children, *Developmental Psychology,* 1973, *9,* 236-245.

Fry, D. Word and sentence tests for use in speech audiometry. *Lancet,* 1961, *22,* 197-199.

Geffen, G., & Sexton, M. The development of auditory strategies of attention. *Developmental Psychology,* 1978, *14,* 11-17.

Goldman, R., Fristoe, M., & Woodcock, R. Test of auditory discrimination, Circle Pines, MN: American Guidance Service, 1970.

Hagen, J. Strategies for remembering. In S. Farnham-Diggory (Ed.), *Information processing in children.* New York: Academic Press, 1972, 65-79.

Halford, G., & Wilson, W. A category theory approach to cognitive development. *Cognitive Psychology,* 1980, *12,* 356-411.

Haskins, H. A phonetically balanced test of speech discrimination for children. Master's thesis, Northwestern University, 1949.

Hirsh, I., Davis, H., Silverman, S., Reynolds, E., Eldert, E., & Benson, R. Development of materials for speech audiometry. *Journal of Speech and Hearing Disorders,* 1952, *17,* 321-337.

Jerger, S. Unpublished data. Baylor College of Medicine, 1980.

Jerger, S., & Jerger, J. Estimating speech threshold from the PI-PB function. *Archives of Otolaryngology,* 1976, *102,* 487-496.

Jerger, S., & Jerger, J. Pediatric speech intelligibility test: Performance—intensity characteristics. *Ear and Hearing,* 1982, *3,* 325-334.

Jerger, S., Jerger, J., & Lewis, S. Pediatric speech intelligibility test. II. Effect of receptive language age and chronological age. *International Journal of Pediatric Otorhinolaryngology,* 1981, *3,* 101-118.

Jerger, S., Lewis, S., Hawkins, J., & Jerger, J. Pediatric speech intelligibility test. I. Generation of test materials. *International Journal of Pediatric Otorhinolaryngology,* 1980, *2,* 217-230.

Keating, D., Keniston, A., Manis, F., & Bobbitt, B. Development of the search-processing parameter. *Child Development,* 1980, *51,* 39-44.

Keith, R. *Central auditory dysfunction.* New York: Grune & Stratton, 1977.

Kelley, B., & Pillow, G. Nonsense syllable discrimination by picture identification with young children. *Journal of the American Auditory Society,* 1979, *4,* 170-172.

Kobasigawa, A. Utilization of retrieval cues by children in recall. *Child Development,* 1974, *45,* 127-134.

Kramer, P., Koff, E., & Fowles, B. Enactment vs. picture-choice tasks in studies of early language comprehension: When a picture is not worth 10,000 words, *Psychological Reports,* 1980, *46,* 803-806.

Lee, L. *The Northwestern Syntax Screening Test.* Evanston, IL: Northwestern University Press, 1971.

Lenel, J., & Cantor, J. Rhyme recognition and phonemic perception in young children, *Journal of Psycholinguistic Research,* 1981, *10,* 57-67.

Luria, A. *The working brain. An introduction to neuropsychology.* New York: Basic Books, 1973, 83-89.

Luszcz, M, & Bacharach, V. Preschoolers' picture recognition memory: The pitfalls of knowing how a thing shall be called. *Canadian Journal of Psychological Review,* 1980, *34,* 155-160.

Marshall, L., Brandt, J., Marston, L., & Ruder, K. Changes in number and type of errors on repetition of acoustically distorted sentences as a function of age in normal children. *Journal of the American Auditory Society,* 1979, *4,* 218-226.

Marslen-Wilson, W., & Welsh, A. Processing interactions and lexical access during word recognition in continuous speech. *Cognitive Psychology,* 1978, *10,* 29-63.

Miller, G., & Johnson-Laird, P. *Language and perception.* Cambridge: Harvard University Press, 1976.

Nagafuchi, N. Intelligibility of distorted speech sounds shifted in frequency and time in normal children. *Audiology,* 1976, *15,* 326-337.

Nelson, N. Comprehension of spoken language by normal children as a function of speaking rate, sentence difficulty, and listener age and sex. *Child Development,* 1976, *47,* 299-303.

Niemeyer, W. Speech audiometry with phonetically balanced sentences, *Audiology,* 1965, *4,* 97-101.

Norman, D. *Memory and attention. An introduction to human information processing* (2nd Ed.) New York: John Wiley, 1976.

Olsen, W., & Matkin, N. Speech audiometry. In W. Rintelmann (Ed.), *Hearing assessment.* Baltimore: University Park Press, 1979, 133-206.

Palva, A., & Jokinen, K. Undistorted and filtered speech audiometry in children with normal hearing. *Acta Otolaryngolica,* 1975, *80,* 383-388.

Rose, D. Some functional correlates of the maturation of neural systems. In D. Caplan (Ed.), *Biological studies of mental processes,* Cambridge: MIT Press, 1980, 27-43.

Ross, M., & Lerman, J. A picture identification test for hearing-impaired children. *Journal of Speech and Hearing Research,* 1970, *13,* 44-53.

Sanderson-Leepa, M., & Rintelmann, W. Articulation functions and test-retest performance of normal-hearing children on three speech discrimination tests: WIPI, PBK-50, and NU auditory test no. 6. *Journal of Speech and Hearing Disorders,* 1976, *41,* 503-519.

Schwartz, A., & Goldman, R. Variables influencing performance on speech-sound discrimination tests. *Journal of Speech and Hearing Research,* 1974, *17,* 25-32.

Siegenthaler, B. Maturation of auditory abilities in children. *Audiology,* 1969, *8,* 59-71.

Siegenthaler, B. Reliability of the TIP and DIP speech-hearing tests for children. *Journal of Communication Disorders,* 1975, *8,* 325-333.

Simon, C., & Fourcin, A. Cross-language study of speech-pattern learning. *Journal of The Acoustical Society of America,* 1978, *63,* 925-935.

Smith, K., & Hodgson, W. The effects of systematic reinforcement on the speech discrimination responses of normal and hearing-impaired children. *Journal of Audiological Research,* 1970, *10,* 110-117.

Speaks, C. Performance-intensity characteristics of selected verbal materials. *Journal of Speech and Hearing Research,* 1967, *10,* 344-347.

Speaks, C., & Jerger, J. Method for measurement of speech identification. *Journal of Speech and Hearing Research,* 1965, *8,* 185-194.

Speaks, C., Jerger, J., & Jerger, S. Performance-intensity characteristics of synthetic sentences. *Journal of Speech and Hearing Research,* 1966, *9,* 305-312.

Speaks, C., Karmen, J., & Benitez, L. Effect of a competing message on synthetic sentence identification. *Journal of Speech and Hearing Research,* 1967, *10,* 390-396.

Teatini, G. Sensitized speech test results in school children. In C. Rojskjaer (Ed.), *Speech audiometry,* Odense, Denmark: Danavox, 1970, 102-111.

Watson, T. Speech audiometry for children. In A. Ewing (Ed.), *Educational guidance and the deaf child.* Washington, DC: The Volta Bureau, 1957, 278-296.

Willeford, J. Assessing central auditory behavior in children: A test battery approach. In R. Keith (Ed.), *Central auditory dysfunction.* New York: Grune & Stratton, 1977, 43-68.

Willeford, J. Expanded central auditory test battery norms. Cited in R. Keith (Ed.), *Central auditory and language disorders in children.* San Diego: College-Hill Press, 1981, 61-76.

Wilson, R., & Antablin, J. A picture identification task as an estimate of the word-recognition performance of nonverbal adults. *Journal of Speech and Hearing Disorders,* 1980, *45,* 223-238.

Zukier, H., & Hagen, J. The development of selective attention under distracting conditions, *Child Development,* 1978, *49,* 870-873.

Don W. Worthington
Jon F. Peters

Electrophysiologic Audiometry

Introduction

Behavioral audiological evaluations are often unsuccessful with un-
cooperative and/or noncommunicative patients. Attempts have been made
to develop objective tests of auditory function for these patients. These
attempts have focused primarily on physiological variables such as the
cochleopalpebral reflex, heart rate, respiration, psychogalvonic skin
response (PGSR), and acoustic reflex and immittance measures (Bradford,
1975; Jerger, 1973). Although each of these tests has shown some degree
of clinical utility, they are generally lacking in their ability to provide site-
of-lesion information.

One technique, the auditory-evoked potential (AEP), seemed particularly
suited to this task. While the initial clinical reports on the AEP were prom-
ising, the within- and between-subject variance was problematical (see
Davis, 1976; for a review). The degradation of the response with sleep (either
sedated or natural), and the poor definition of the response near threshold
were major sources of error. These problems were particularly evident when
the technique was applied to pediatric cases, especially multiply handicapped and noncommunicative patients. Despite these shortcomings, the late
components (N_1, P_2) laid the background for the AEP as an objective
test of auditory sensitivity. Goldstein and his colleagues subsequently
published a series of papers on the "early" —now generally referred to
as the "middle"— components of the AEP (Mendel & Goldstein, 1969a,

1969b, 1971). These components, which occur in the time frame of 20-80 msecs after stimulus onset, were reported to be relatively state independent, stable across subjects, and identifiable near threshold. Although the clinical application of these components was delayed by concerns over their origin, the middle response has demonstrable audiological and neurological applications (Mendel, 1978; Ozdamar, Kvaus, & Curvy, 1982; Vivion, 1980).

Recently, Galambos, Makeig, and Talmachoff (1981) demonstrated that by compounding the middle components through fast (≈ 40/sec) stimulus rates, behavioral thresholds for low frequency tones could be approximated.

In 1971, Jewett and Williston described a set of early components of the AEP in man which occurred in the first 10 msec following stimulus onset. They considered this response to be a reflection of the electrical activity of the auditory pathways of the brainstem. Similar components had been described by Sohmer and Feinmesser (1967) and Yoshie (1968) in their studies on electrocochleography. This response, currently referred to as the auditory brainstem response (ABR), has become a cornerstone of objective audiometry for difficult-to-test patients. The ABR is stable both within and between subjects, either awake, asleep, or sedated, and approximates behavioral thresholds for the higher frequencies (Jerger & Mauldin, 1978). Although the clinical acceptance of the technique was slow, it is now an important diagnostic tool in the armementarium of the audiologist, otolaryngologist, and neurologist (see Fria, 1980; Rowe, 1981; Stockard, Stockard, & Sharbrough, 1978; Stockard, Stockard, Westmoreland, & Corfits, 1979; for reviews).

The following sections, based on data collected at the Boys Town Institute, illustrate the application of the ABR in the audiometric assessment of pediatric populations.

Interpretative Guidelines

Once the complex interactions between recording, stimulus, and patient variables are understood (Picton, Woods, & Baribeau-Braun, 1977; Stockard, Stockard, & Sharbrough, 1978; Stockard, Stockard, Westmoreland, & Corfits, 1979), and a population-specific normative data base has been established, interpretative guidelines are necessary. Figure 4-1 depicts our guidelines, which are similar to those outlined by Despland and Galambos (1980).

If the absolute latencies (AL) and relative amplitudes (RA) of Waves I and V are both normal and the I-V interpeak latency (IPL) is also normal, then a neurological disorder is unlikely. If responses are evident at least down to 30 dB HL, then a major peripheral auditory deficit is unlikely. When the AL of Waves I and V is prolonged, but the I-V IPL is normal,

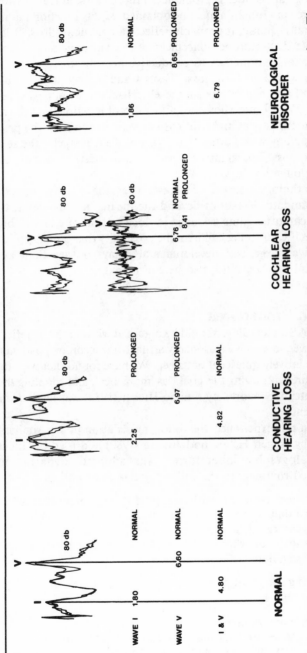

FIGURE 4-1
ABRs Obtained From Four Infants Referred From the Intensive Care Nursery

NOTE: These waveforms are typical of those recorded from patients in each of the four categories. The following parameters were used to record these and all other ABRs presented in this text. N = 1024, gain = 100K, Bandpass = 100 - 3000 Hz, Rarefaction clicks were presented at 11.8 per second.

an audiological disorder is probable. In those cases, at least a three-point latency-intensity function must be obtained. If this function parallels that of a normal response, it probably reflects a conductive loss. It is important to note that improper placement of the earphone and/or collapsing ear canals can masquerade as conductive hearing loss.

In cases with a cochlear loss, Waves I and V may occur with normal AL and IPLs at higher intensity levels. However, as intensity decreases, the AL to Wave V may show a significant prolongation; and the response may be evident only at higher intensity levels. In addition, the probability of recording any waves other than Wave V decreases with the severity of the cochlear loss. Several intensity levels must be tested to resolve the cause of the prolongation in Wave V.

Neuropathology is suspected in cases where the IPLs are more than two or three standard deviations beyond the mean. In some cases, this prolongation can offer some evidence for localization of a lesion, but is not disease specific. In young children, the possibility that prolonged IPLs may be reflective of general developmental delays, rather than an active pathological process, must also be considered.

Sedation Procedures

Ideally, ABR recordings should be obtained without the benefit of sedation. However, to assure a reasonably artifact-free recording, patients should be either relatively quiescent or asleep. We have found that with difficult-to-test children, achieving this goal was impractical, and adopting the "wait-'em-out" attitude favored by Finitzo-Hieber (1982) was neither time- nor cost-efficient.

Based on this experience, the following sedation policy, similar to that described by Jerger, Hayes, and Jordan (1980) and used in clinical electroencephalographic laboratories, was adopted. Sedation may be administered routinely to the following classes of patients:

1. Patients over 12 months of age if it is apparent that artifact-free recordings cannot be obtained without sedation, and in the absence of contraindications.
2. Patients for whom the referring physician has requested the use of sedation.

The following classes of patients are not sedated unless authorized by the referring physician:

1. Pregnant women.
2. Patients with indicated renal or hepatic failure.
3. Outpatients who come to the laboratory unaccompanied.

The sedation of choice is chloral hydrate (40-60 mg/kg of body weight with a maximum of 1 gm per single dose). It is administered orally, in liquid form. The action of this drug is confined principally to the cerebral hemispheres. Blood pressure and respiration are depressed only slightly more than in normal sleep. Reflexes are not significantly depressed. The initial dose of medication is administered 15 minutes before the recording is started. Resedation (50% of the original dose) is considered if there is no sign of drowsiness within 30 minutes and administered only if the physician in charge concurs.

In cases where chloral hydrate is not effective, a "lytic cocktail, " an intramuscular injection of Demerol, Phenegran, and Thorazine (2:1:1 mg/kg respectively), is considered. This sedative presents a greater risk than chloral hydrate, and the patient must be monitored carefully. Its use is contraindicated in cases who have experienced a previous allergic or adverse reaction to any of the three component drugs and/or individuals on monoamine oxidase inhibitors.

When necessary, general anesthesia can be utilized without affecting the ABR results (Duncan, Sanders, & McCullough, 1979: Sanders, Duncan, & McCullough, 1979; Stockard et al., 1978). It must be emphasized that the use of sedation is a medical procedure and must be done with proper safeguards and medical supervision.

Table 4-1 summarizes our experience with this sedation philosophy. Oral administration of chloral hydrate was effective in 61.5% of the total patients on initial administration, with 87.2% of all patients being examined successfully following a second dose (one-half the initial dose after 30-45 minutes). A lytic cocktail was always effective on first administration. Valium was not effective in most cases and its use was discontinued. The relatively high incidence of the use of general anesthesia was related to the performance of myringotomies prior to the ABR evaluation. For those patients, the evaluation was completed at surgery as a matter of convenience. For the remaining 2.8% of the patients, no other form of sedation was effective. In fact, reviews of their medical charts revealed that previous attempts at sedation for other diagnostic procedures were unsuccessful. These data agree with those of Jerger, Hayes, and Jordan (1980), and support chloral hydrate as an effective sedative for ABR evaluations.

Intensive Care Nursery

Perhaps the best-known application of the ABR is in the screening of intensive care nursery (ICN) graduates (Hecox & Galambos, 1974; Mokotoff, Schulman-Galambos, & Galambos, 1977; Schulman-Galambos & Galambos, 1975). The ABR abnormalities seen in ICN survivors can

TABLE 4-1
Percentage of Cases Within Each Group of Patients Receiving Various Sedation Regimes

	Mental retardation	Developmental delays	Down's syndrome
Sedation not necessary	3.0	1.4	12.5
Sedated once—chloral hydrate	40.6	71.0	37.5
Sedated twice—chloral hydrate	37.5	20.3	25.0
Sedated once—lytic cocktail	6.3	4.4	0
Sedated once—valium	4.8	0	11.2
Sedation not effective	1.5	0	1.3
General anesthesia	6.3	2.9	12.5

be divided into two general categories, those presumed to reflect neuropathology and those presumed to reflect the presence of hearing loss. This categorization is dictated in part by the reported incidence of ABR abnormalities, which ranges from estimates of 9 to approximately 37% (Amlie, Sanders, Huxtable, & Starr, 1978) as compared to the incidence of significant hearing loss in ICN graduates which varies from approximately 5% to 25% (Table 4-2). Cox, Hack, and Metz, (1981a, 1981b) accounted for at least a portion of this discrepancy on the basis of interlaboratory procedural differences. For example, some investigators obtained responses only at 60 dB HL and defined an abnormal ABR on the basis of Wave V latency only. The statistical definition of an abnormal peak latency varies between one and two standard deviations beyond the mean. The incidence of ABR abnormalities will vary greatly on the basis of this definition alone. Part of the variability in the reported data can be attributed to the interaction between intensity level, rate of stimulus presentation, click polarity, and patient age (Stockard & Westmoreland, 1981).

Several investigators (Despland & Galambos, 1980; Schulman-Galambos & Galambos, 1979a, 1979b) report only the number of infants suspected to have a sensorineural hearing loss, while others collapse the sensorineural and conductive hearing-loss cases along with all other ABR abnormalities into one category (Mjoen, 1981; Wilson, 1982).

In addition, the physiological status of the infants has varied from those tested at 4 days of age while confined to isolettes in the ICN, to older, healthier infants confined to the ICN, but breathing room air. Still others were tested at discharge in audiometric sound suites. The contribution of

TABLE 4-2
Estimated Incidence of Hearing Loss in Intensive Care Nursery Patients Based on ABR Results

Investigators	Reported Incidence (%)
Schulman-Galambos & Galambos (1979)	5.3
Despland & Galambos (1980)	8–12
Marshall, Reichert, Kerley, & Davis (1980)	9
Cox & Metz (1980); Cox, Hack, & Metz (1981a)	5–9
Wilson (1982)	20
Mjoen (1981)	25

this variance in physiological status to the incidence of ABR abnormalities is difficult to assess.

Although Marshall, Reichert, Kerley, and Davis (1980) and Stockard and Westmoreland (1981) alluded to the possibility that the background noise level in the ICN may effect the ABR, most investigators have ignored this variable. Some reported that the background noise level was not sufficient to affect the ABR threshold for adults. Others have corrected for the noise level by setting click intensity relative to adult behavioral thresholds obtained in the ICN. The assumption is that the background noise levels encountered in the ICN will have the same effect on the response of a neonate as it would on the response of a normal adult. To our knowledge, this assumption is not supported in the literature. In addition, the possibility that infants tested in isolettes may be experiencing a temporary threshold shift must also be considered. That adults with cochlear losses respond differently in environments with different levels of background noise is well known.

Another possible source of variance is the potential for error in determining the infant's gestational age. For example, the accuracy of these tests varies with the time assessment relative to the neonate's birth and the physiological status of the mother at delivery. Most tests are considered to be accurate within a range of 1 to 2 weeks. However, the 95% confidence level is generally stated as plus or minus 2 weeks. Thus, there is a possibility of at least a 2-week error in the estimation of gestational age. Since the ABR can undergo rapid, significant changes in latency, amplitude, and threshold over a 1 to 4 week time span in early life, the error variance is obvious.

In order to minimize the role of these variables, we conduct the ABR evaluations only when the infant is healthy and breathing room air. Further constraints are the absence of any evidence of respiratory distress, systemic illness, apnea, or bradycardia. The infants exhibit good feeding status and are ready for discharge at the time of the ABR exam. All evaluations are carried out in a sound suite.

Table 4-3 summarizes our results collected from 225 infants referred from one ICN over a 2-year period. Approximately 64% of the infants were considered to have normal peripheral auditory sensitivity in each ear and no evidence of neuropathology. An additional 15% appeared to have normal peripheral sensitivity in at least one ear, while 21% showed abnormal results in both ears. Table 4-4 shows the percentage of infants whose ABRs were judged to be reflective of a hearing loss (conductive, sensorineural, or mixed) and neuropathology/neural maturational delays.

Of the 16% suspected of having a bilateral hearing loss, initial evaluation indicated that 12% were conductive, 2% cochlear, and 2% mixed. Unilateral hearing loss was noted in 12%. If these two groups are combined, then 5% of the infants showed cochlear involvement. These results are consistent with those reported by Schulman-Galambos and Galambos (1979b), Marshall et al. (1980), Despland and Galambos (1980), and Cox et al. (1981a). A total of 25% were suspected of having a conductive hearing loss. This percentage is consistent with the reported incidence of middle ear effusion in infants in ICNs (Balkany, Berman, Simmons, & JaFek, 1978; Schaffer & Angell, 1977).

Infants whose ABRs were suggestive of the presence of neuropathology and/or maturational delays in the auditory pathways (Table 4-4) exhibited bilateral or unilateral IPLs greater than two standard deviations beyond the mean. The category of "neural maturational delays" was added, as similar prolonged IPLs have been noted in older children who exhibit severe developmental, speech, and language delays. Unfortunately, we cannot differentiate infants within this broad category. If the infant ABR is predictive of developmental delays, identification using this technique could be followed by early intervention. This approach is supported, in part, by the data of Salamy, Mendelson, Tooley, and Chaplin (1980a, 1980b), which showed significant differences in the ABRs of healthy and high-risk infants up to 1 year of age.

Since the ABR is sensitive to both pathological and maturational changes affecting the auditory pathways, follow-up evaluations are a must for any infant in whom an abnormal ABR is found. The following case emphasized this need.

J. D. was delivered by C-section following premature rupture of the membrane at an estimated gestational age of 32-33 weeks. Birth weight was

TABLE 4-3
Percentage of Normal and Abnormal ABR Findings in 225 Neonates Referred from the ICN. Audiological and Neurological Abnormalities Have Been Combined in the Cells Labeled Abnormal.

		Right Ear	
		Normal	Abnormal
Left Ear	Normal	64%	6%
	Abnormal	9%	21%

TABLE 4-4
Percentage of Abnormal ABRs Divided Into Specific Diagnostic Categories

	Normal %	Conductive %	Sensori-neural %	Mixed %	Neuropathology and/or Neural Maturational Delays %
Normal	64	11	1	0	2
Conductive		12	0	0	3*
Sensorineural			2	0	2*
Mixed				2	0
Neuropathology and/or Neural Maturational Delays					10*

*Contains children with combination of hearing loss and neuropathology.

4 pounds, 9 ounces, with Apgars of 7 and 7 at 1 and 5 minutes, respectively. Respiratory distress syndrome, with mild asphyxia and hypotension, was also noted. His progress was satisfactory and he was considered ready for discharge at 19 days of age. The ABR completed just prior to discharge is shown in Figure 4-2. Stimulation of the left ear at 80 dB HL elicited an ABR consisting of Waves I, III, and V with prolonged interwave and Wave V latencies. This response was replicable down to 60 dB HL with a prolonged Wave V latency. Stimulation of the right ear at 80 dB HL elicited an ABR consisting of Waves I, II, III, and V with prolonged interwave and Wave V latencies. This response was replicable down to 40 dB HL with prolonged Wave V latency-intensity function. A moderate high-frequency loss on the left, and a mild-to-moderate high-frequency loss on

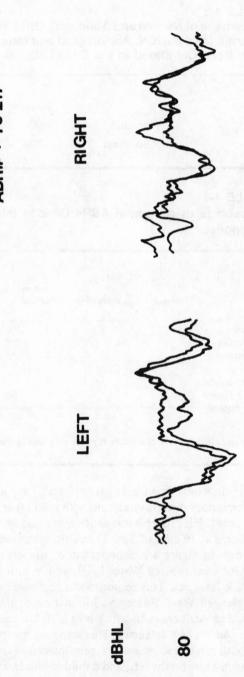

FIGURE 4-2
ABRs Recorded on J. D. at Discharge From the ICN

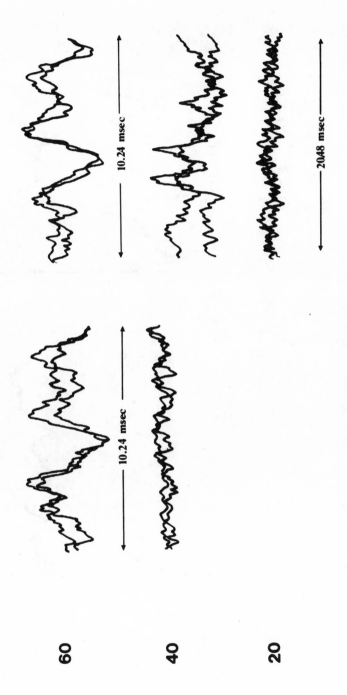

FIGURE 4-3
ABRs Recorded at Follow-Up—6 Months After Those Seen in Figure 4-2

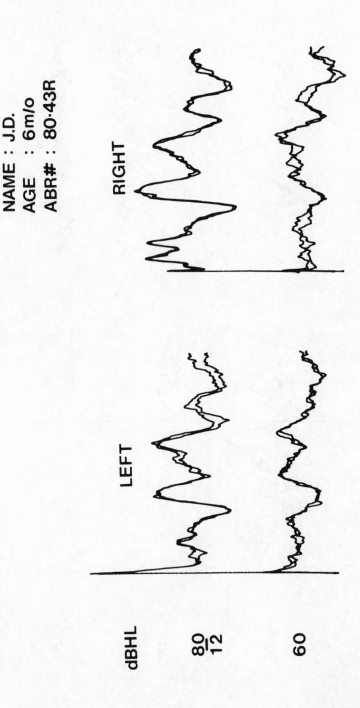

NAME : J.D.
AGE   : 6m/o
ABR# : 80·43R

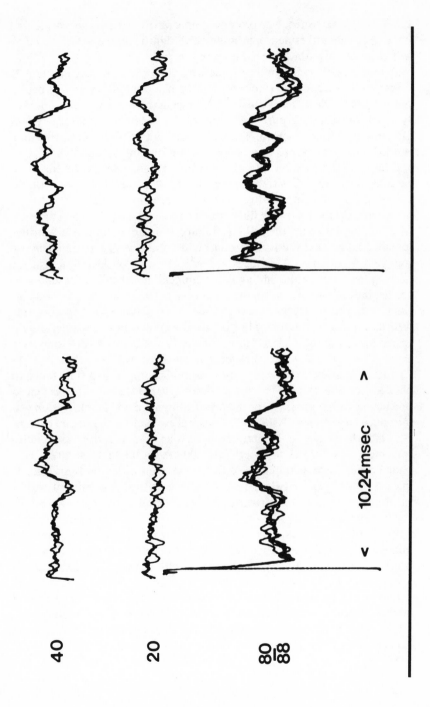

the right was suspected. The prolonged interwave latencies were considered consistent with either neuropathology or a significant maturational delay in the auditory pathways of the brainstem.

A repeat ABR evaluation at 6 months of age is shown in Figure 4-3. These responses show no evidence of either neuropathology and/or neural maturational delays. The significant change in the Wave V latency intensity function, seen in Figure 4-4, supported a peripheral auditory system functioning within the normal range of sensitivity. Subsequent behavioral audiological evaluations confirmed normal hearing bilaterally.

Although the number of infants who demonstrate improvement in peripheral auditory sensitivity in the absence of a conductive loss is small, the need for follow-up testing cannot be overemphasized.

In contrast, the following illustrates a case in which early identification of a hearing loss with the ABR facilitated the habilitation of a hearing-impaired infant. R. M. was the product of a normal pregnancy and delivery, weighing 6 pounds, 11¼ ounces at birth. He was considered at risk for hearing loss, as an older sibling had a congenital severe-to-profound sensorineural hearing loss of unknown etiology. The ABR completed on R. M. at 5 days of age is shown in Figure 4-5. No replicable ABR components were seen following monaural or binaural stimulation at any intensity up to and including 102 dB HL. Since no neurological signs or symptoms were evident, the ABR data was considered as consistent with a profound, high-frequency hearing loss bilaterally. Behavioral testing at that time failed to elicit any responses, even to intense stimuli (110 dB HL). R. M. was placed in a parent-infant program for the hearing impaired and amplification was introduced after repeat ABR and behavioral evaluations showed no change. By 7 months of age, behavioral responses were obtained with Visual Reinforcement Audiometry to speech and 500 Hz warble tones at 90 dB HL. Aided results demonstrated good functional gain with a body-style hearing aid. Subsequent ABR evaluations continued to be consistent with a profound, bilateral, high-frequency sensorineural loss. Figure 4-6 shows the audiogram obtained on R. M. at 2 years of age, which is consistent with the interpretation of the ABRs, indicating the presence of a profound bilateral, high-frequency cochlear loss. In this case, early identification of hearing loss by the ABR was corroborated with behavioral and impedance results.

Our results support the use of ABR audiometry to assess the peripheral auditory status of newborn infants. If the ABR can be shown to be predictive of other handicapping conditions, as well as hearing deficits, then the expenditure of time and money would be more than justifiable.

FIGURE 4-4
**Wave V Latency Intensity Functions for the ABRs Seen in Figures
4-2 and 4-3**

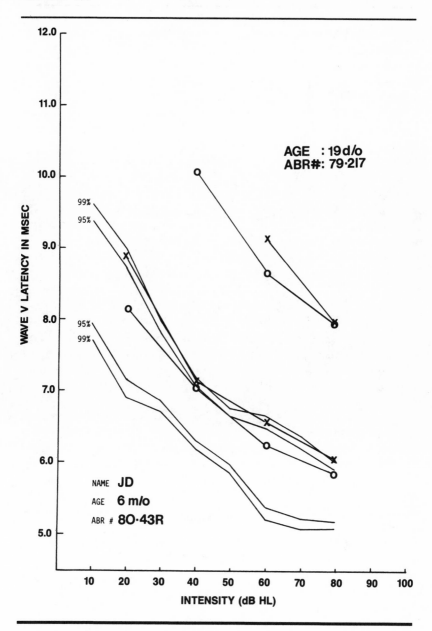

FIGURE 4-5
ABRs Recorded on RM at 5 Days of Age

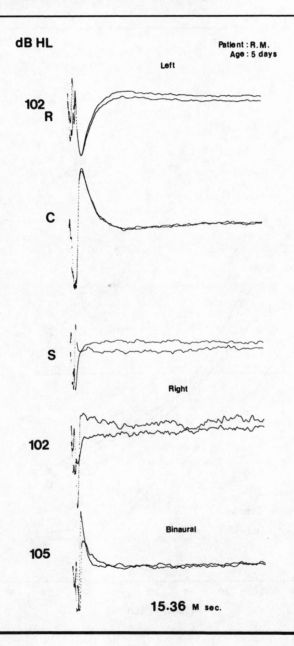

FIGURE 4-6
Audiogram Obtained on RM at 2 Years of Age

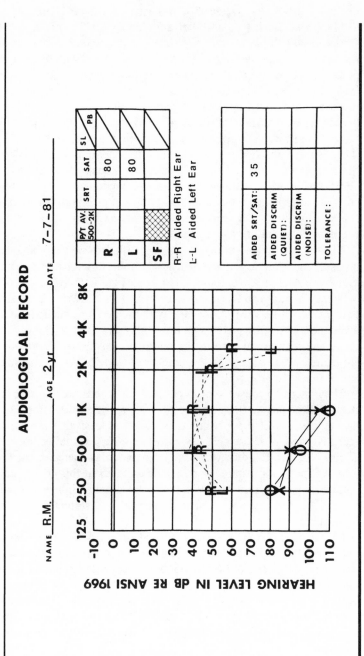

Developmental, Speech, and Language Delays

Tallal and Stark (1981), Tallal and Piercy (1973a, 1973b, 1974), and Frumkin and Rapin (1980) have shown that language-impaired children perform significantly poorer on auditory discrimination tasks that incorporate brief temporal cues, when compared to children with normal language. Their ability to respond correctly to rapidly presented verbal materials was also impaired relative to that of normal children. They hypothesized that these performance deficits might be related, at least in part, to a primary auditory perceptual deficit in temporal analysis. Since the ABR is considered to reflect timing or temporal processing in the brainstem auditory pathways (Galambos & Hecox, 1978; Starr & Achor, 1975), asymmetries in the latency-intensity function and/or prolonged IPLs could be interpreted as being reflective of disrupted peripheral timing processes. Thus, the ABR seemed the logical tool to test their hypothesis in the peripheral auditory system.

ABRs were obtained from two groups of children who exhibited language and speech or developmental delays. The following ABR parameters were evaluated: ALs of Waves I and V, IPLs of Waves I-III, III-V, and I-V, Wave V latency-intensity functions, symmetry of IPL and Wave V ALs, and the agreement of the Wave V threshold with the audiometric threshold (when available). The ABR and impedance data were used to classify each ear as reflecting normal peripheral auditory sensitivity; conductive, sensorineural, or mixed hearing loss; and/or neuropathology or neural maturational delays.

The first group consisted of 18 children with moderate-to-severe language delays. They ranged in age from 28 to 62 months with a median age of 44 months. All of these children exhibited at least an 8-month delay in receptive and/or expressive language, and 92% exhibited more than a 12-month delay. Children with mild language delays were excluded to avoid a high false-negative rate. None of the children in this group had a sensorineural hearing loss, based on their behavioral audiometric results, and all had normal intelligence when assessed with standard nonverbal intelligence test.

Of the 18 children, five were normal on all ABR measures and five demonstrated ABR results consistent with conductive hearing loss. Of the remaining eight cases (44.4%), poor agreement between the ABR threshold and the audiometric threshold was noted in two, one demonstrated prolonged IPLs bilaterally, asymmetries in IPLs exceeding 0.3 millisecond were seen in three, and the latency intensity functions were significantly asymmetrical in two cases, even though the IPLs were within normal limits for each ear.

The incidence of ABR abnormalities in this initial population prompted us to review the ABR data collected on patients previously referred to the Institute for evaluation of significant speech, language, and developmental delays who had no prior diagnosis of hearing loss. This review yielded the 180 cases described in Table 4-5. Of these, 52 were found to have normal peripheral auditory sensitivity and no ABR abnormalities, 12 had conductive hearing impairments bilaterally, 41 showed bilateral cochlear impairment, and 12 demonstrated bilateral, mixed impairments. Thirty-five cases exhibited results consistent with bilateral neuropathology and/or neuromaturational delays in the auditory pathways of the brainstem. Ten cases with normal peripheral sensitivity showed asymmetrical IPLs of at least 0.3 milliseconds.

In summary, 25% of the cases in the second group demonstrated ABR abnormalities that were consistent with the presence of neuropathology or maturational delays in the auditory pathways of the brainstem. This compares to the 44% noted in the first group. This difference between the findings in the two groups is attributed to the broad diagnostic categories, including mental retardation, in the second group.

The cases reported here represent a heterogeneous group of children exhibiting speech and language delays. Although the distribution of ABR abnormalities is not the same for the two groups, we suspect that they may be reflective of a similar process. Further investigation is required to determine if the subtle differences in neural transmission time, as reflected in the ABR data, can predict the disruption of normal speech and language development.

Other investigators have used similar findings in patients exhibiting hereditary motor-sensory neuropathy, autism, and spastic dysphonia (Satya-Murti, Cacace, & Hanson, 1979; Sharbrough, Stockard, & Aronson, 1978; Student & Sohmer, 1978) to argue for the presence of organic lesions or maturational delays in the auditory pathways of the brainstem.

Multiply Handicapped/Mentally Retarded/Autistic

In applying the ABR to multiply handicapped, autistic, and retarded patients, the presence or absence of central nervous system (CNS) pathology can affect the outcome of the evaluation (Jerger, Hayes, & Jordan, 1980; Jerger, Neely, & Jerger, 1980; Skoff, Mirsky, & Turner, 1980). However, once this limit is identified, the ABR remains the best measure presently available for objectively evaluating the auditory status in these populations. Unfortunately, the audiometric application of the ABR in severely handicapped older populations is not well documented, as the majority of

TABLE 4-5
Categorization of the ABR Results in Children with Severe Speech and Language Delays

	Normal	Conductive	Sensori-neural	Mixed	Neuropathology/ Maturational Delay
Normal	52	3	6	1	10
Conductive		12	1	1	1
Sensorineural			41	2	3
Mixed				12	0
Neuropathology/ Maturational Delay					35

investigations have focused on the detection of subtle CNS pathology (Edwards, Tanguay, Schwafel, Norman, Squires, & Buchwald, 1980; Ornitz & Walter, 1975; Skoff et al., 1980; Sohmer & Student, 1978; Squires, Aine, Buchwald, Norman, & Galbraith, 1980; Student & Sohmer, 1978). Several of these reports did, however, note a relatively high incidence of hearing loss in the populations studied. In contrast, Peters, Beauchaine, Reiland, and Worthington (1981) reported on the relative incidence of hearing loss as defined by the ABR within a severely handicapped population. Their selective review of 800 patients seen for ABR evaluations offered the populations shown in Table 4-6. Although all of these patients exhibited some degree of mental retardation, they were grouped according to the presence/absence of that diagnosis in their medical history. Further analysis within each group did not reveal any one medical problem to be predominant in any group. The most common problem was a seizure disorder, with cerebral palsy and micro- or hydrocephalus also prominent. The patients were generally older and usually were referred from long-term care facilities. Because of the limited sample size, no attempt was made to analyze the data according to sex or age, either within or between these groups. At least 40% of the patients were found to have some form of external ear canal blockage which required removal prior to the ABR evaluation. Tympanometric evaluations were carried out on all patients with suspected middle ear dysfunction.

The data from each group were divided into five categories of hearing loss on the basis of the lowest intensity level at which a replicable Wave V could be recorded regardless of latency. As can be seen in Table 4-7, the percentage of individuals with hearing loss varied widely in the three

TABLE 4-6
Characteristics of the Three Populations Reviewed

	Medical Complications		Sex		Age[a]
	Yes	*No*	*M*	*F*	
Mental retardation	21	11	20	12	13.5 (2–40)
Developmental delays	29	40	43	26	3.4 (1–13)
Down's syndrome	2	6	5	3	8.5 (1-30)

Note: These cases reflect 13.6% of the last 800 cases seen.
[a]Numbers in parentheses indicate the age range of the patients within each group.

groups. In the majority (76.4%) of patients exhibiting a hearing loss, the loss was asymmetrical. In the four patients from whom no ABR could be recorded, the possibility of retrocochlear involvement could not be ruled out. In the remainder of the patients, however, the overall Wave V latency-intensity functions were considered to be within the range expected for a hearing loss of the degree inferred from the Wave V threshold.

Of the 57 patients showing some degree of hearing loss, 49.1% were judged to be of cochlear origin. The remainder were classified as either conductive (13.2%) or a combination of cochlear and conductive (37.7%). Unfortunately, it is difficult to distinguish the mixed losses from retrocochlear involvement because often Wave I is absent.

Due to the difficulty encountered in testing these patients with behavioral techniques, audiometric data was available on only 13. Comparison of the behavioral and ABR data for these patients showed, at worst, a 20 dB discrepancy between the Wave V threshold and the average behavioral threshold at 1, 2, and 4 KHz for any single patient. These findings are in good agreement with the data reported by Sohoel, Mair, Elverland, and Laukli (1979).

ABR in Post-Meningitic Children

The incidence of hearing loss in children recovering from meningitis has been studied extensively. The reported incidence of hearing loss in children

TABLE 4-7
Percentage of Cases Showing Symmetrical and Asymmetrical Hearing Losses in Each Population

Mental Retardation dB HL[a]	Normal	Mild	Moderate	Severe	Profound
20–30 Normal	4.3	3.1	3.1	0	0
40–50 Mild		12.5	12.5	3.1	0
60–70 Moderate			6.3	0	6.3
80 Severe			0	0	0
90 Profound					18.8
Developmental Delay					
Normal	58.0	7.2	0	0	1.4
Mild		4.3	4.3	1.4	0
Moderate			8.7	4.7	4.3
Severe			0	0	1.4
Profound					4.3
Down's Syndrome					
Normal	12.5	12.5	0	0	0
Mild		37.5	0	0	0
Moderate			25.0	0	0
Severe			0	0	0
Profound					12.5

[a]db HL indicates the lowest intensity level at which a Wave V could be recorded.

secondary to meningitis ranges from 5% to 35%. The sooner the presence of a hearing loss can be diagnosed, the better the prognosis for alleviating at least some of the psychological and educational delays frequently experienced by hearing-impaired children (Nylen & Rosenhall, 1979; Vernon, 1967). The diagnosis of hearing loss is a particular problem in postmeningitic populations due to their relatively young age and the frequent presence of compounding neuropsychological sequelae (Rosenhall & Kankkunen, 1980). This population would appear to be suited to evaluation with the ABR, which has been successful in the evaluation of kernicterus infants (Chisin, Perlman, & Sohmer, 1979; Kaga, Kitazumi, & Kodama, 1979), perinatal asphyxia (Kileny, Connelly, & Robertson, 1980) and high-risk infants as discussed previously.

Kotagal, Rosenberg, Rudd, Dunkle, and Horenstein (1981) demonstrated the feasibility of evaluating post-meningitis cases with the ABR. However, they did not attempt to define the degree of hearing loss in their population. In contrast, Peters and Worthington (1981) and Finitzo-Hieber, Simhadri, and Hieber (1981) reported the incidence of hearing loss as defined by the ABR threshold of Wave V and the shape of the latency-intensity function. The degree of loss suggested by the ABR was confirmed by behavioral data when available.

The original study by Peters and Worthington (1981) has been expanded to include ABR and impedance data from 103 children recovering from meningitis. Based on these results, 43% of the patients exhibited findings consistent with hearing loss, either conductive, mixed, or sensorineural. The ABR thresholds indicated that 65% of these losses were in the severe-to-profound category. These results confirm our previous study and are consistent with the findings of Finitzo-Hieber et al. (1981). None of the cases with presumed cochlear loss showed evidence of recovery on subsequent evaluations. Although abnormally long IPLs were seen frequently in those cases exhibiting significant neurological sequelae, no direct correlations could be made with specific neurological sequelae.

Behavioral Results and No ABR

The principal limitation in the audiologic application of the ABR to a noncommunicative population is the possible presence of CNS pathology (Jerger, Hayes, & Jordan, 1980; Jerger, Neely, & Jerger, 1980). This problem is illustrated in those patients who have normal or near-normal pure-tone thresholds, no demonstrable CNS involvement, and no replicable ABRs (Worthington & Peters, 1980).

R. S. is a 9-year-old female who has significant delays in oral expressive and receptive language and poor visual-motor coordination. She scores in the high average-superior range on nonverbal intelligence tests, with superior visual processing and memory. Her pre- and postnatal history is unremarkable, except for a tonsillectomy and placement of typanostomy tubes at age 3 years. A neurological evaluation at that time suggested possible parietal malfunctions. At the age of 6, she was diagnosed as having congenital aphasia. Repeated audiological assessments showed results ranging from normal to severely impaired hearing. Eventually, conditioned play audiometry, carried out under tight visual and motor structuring, yielded repeatable audiometric data, as seen in Figure 4-7. The tympanograms were normal bilaterally, but the stapedial reflexes were absent at all frequencies at 120 dB HL. Temporal bone tomograms were normal bilaterally. ABR evaluations were carried out on two occasions. The results were identical

FIGURE 4-7
Audiometric and ABR Results for RS

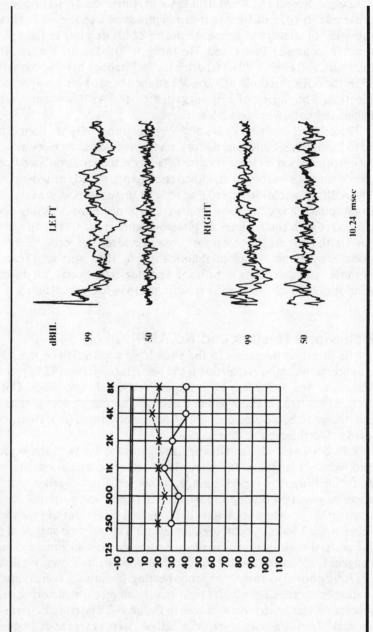

on both tests, with no replicable ABR components elicited with stimulation of either ear at intensity levels up to and including 99 dB HL.

Davis and Hirsh (1979) reported that they have been unable to detect ABR responses in five children who gave "clear evidence of awareness to sound at moderate or quite low intensities." Other investigators have described similar findings (Davis, 1981; Jerger, 1981, personal communication).

Other published reports about the inability to record at least Wave V of the ABR in patients with quantifiable hearing have been confined to patients with demonstrable neurological diseases such as multiple sclerosis. Those reports focused on the dependency of the ABR on the synchronous firing of the eighth nerve and subsequent neurons within the auditory pathway.

Several hypotheses, including (1) absence of neural activity, (2) blocking of nerve conduction, or (3) asynchrony and/or disruption of synchrony have been argued to account for this type of data (Naunton & Fernandez, 1978). The latter hypothesis, asynchrony of discharges in the eighth nerve, may be supported with data from patients with multiple sclerosis who have normal or near-normal audiograms and absent or abnormal ABRs. This suggests that selective demyelinization, lack of myelin formation, and/or neurochemical dysfunction at synaptic junctions in the auditory pathway could be responsible for the asynchrony. In contrast, Davis and Hirsh (1979) suggested that a cochlear impairment could result in sufficient asynchrony to obliterate the ABR. Picton (1978) has also recognized the possibility "that certain auditory nerve or brainstem disorders might interfere with the pathways necessary for the generation of Wave V, and yet leave other pathways that might still provide some 'hearing.'"

As behavioral responses have been noted in patients with no ABR and no known neurological involvement, caution must be exercised in utilizing the ABR as the sole assessment of auditory function. This same caution must be exercised in the presence of a neurological disorder where the absence of an ABR is not necessarily indicative of peripheral auditory dysfunction. The importance of behavioral evaluation and follow-up cannot be overstated, especially when dealing with children.

Neurological Problems

The efficacy of the ABR in the evaluation of patients with suspected neurological diseases is well documented (Robinson & Rudge, 1977; Rowe, 1981; Sohmer, Feinmesser, & Szabo, 1974; Starr & Achor, 1975; Starr & Hamilton, 1976; Stockard & Rossiter, 1977; Stockard, Stockard, & Sharbrough, 1977). However, as Hecox, Cone, and Blaw (1981) noted, only a limited number of these studies dealt with pediatric neurologic applications per se.

Hecox et al. (1981) demonstrated that the ABR can be valuable in the detection and localization of neurological disease in pediatric cases. They concluded:

> The high association between peripheral auditory disorders and neurological abnormalities mandates that both central and peripheral auditory systems receive a full evaluation in the preverbal patient. (p. 839)

Thus, the ABR should be used as part of a battery of tests, especially in the evaluation of the very young and/or difficult-to-test child. Peripheral effects (e.g., conductive hearing loss, severe high-frequency cochlear hearing loss) must be ruled out before an abnormal ABR can be interpreted as indicative of neuropathlogy affecting the auditory pathway of the brainstem.

ABR and Hearing Aid Performance

The possibility of using the ABR to assess hearing aid performance was initially discussed by Picton (1978) and Cox and Metz (1980). More recently, Kileny (1982) concluded that by comparing unaided and aided ABR thresholds, the functional gain provided by a hearing aid could be estimated. Although this technique holds considerable promise for the evaluation of noncommunicative patients, there are a number of technical problems. For example, clicks can cause a large electromagnetic artifact and considerable transient distortion. On the other hand, as Kileny (1982) pointed out, tone pips can induce ringing lasting up to 20 msec, which will affect the identification of any ABR components. Perhaps with additional research and clinical experience, the ABR may be used as a means of determining hearing aid performance.

Summary

It has been demonstrated that the ABR may have both neurological and audiological applications. To this, we would add the possiblity that it may also be reflective of significant maturational delays. Thus, the ABR evaluation should not be considered as a stand-alone objective test of either auditory function or for the detection of neuropathology. Rather, each ABR evaluation must be approached relative to the complete clinical picture of each patient. Similarly, the interpretation must be made in light of that complete picture.

Acknowledgment

The authors express their appreciation to Ms. Jan K. Reiland and Ms. Kathryn A. Beauchaine for their assistance in the collection and tabulation of the data.

References

Amlie, R. N., Sanders, S., Huxtable, R. F., & Starr, A. Objective auditory screening in newborns by auditory brainstem responses (ABR). *Clinical Research*, 1978, *26*, 122A.

Balkany, T. J., Berman, S. A., Simmons, M. A., & JaFek, B. W. Middle ear effusions in neonates. *Laryngoscope*, 1978, *88*, 398–405.

Bradford, L. J. (Ed.). *Physiological measures of the audio-vestibular system*. New York: Academic Press, 1975.

Chisin, R., Perlman, M., & Sohmer, H. Cochlear and brainstem responses in hearing loss following neonatal hyperbilirubinemia. *Annals of Otology*, 1979, *88*, 352–357.

Cox, C., Hack, M., & Metz, D. Brainstem-evoked response audiometry: Normative data from the preterm infant. *Audiology*, 1981, *20*, 53–64. (a)

Cox, C., Hack, M., & Metz, D. A. Brainstem evoked response audiometry in the premature infant population. *International Journal of Pediatric Otorhinolaryngology*, 1981, *3*, 213–224. (b)

Cox, L. C., & Metz, D. ABER in the prescription of hearing aids. *Hearing Instruments*, 1980, *31* (9), 12–15.

Davis, H. Principles of electric response audiometry. *Annals of Otology, Rhinology and Laryngology*, 1976, *85*, 1–96.

Davis, H., & Hirsh, S. K. A slow brainstem response for low-frequency audiometry. *Audiology*, 1979, *18*, 445–461.

Despland, P. A., & Galambos, R. The auditory brainstem response (ABR) is a useful diagnostic tool in the intensive care nursery. *Pediatric Research*, 1980, *14* (2), 154–158.

Duncan, P. G., Sanders, R. A., & McCullough, D. W. Preservation of auditory-evoked brainstem responses in anaesthetized children. *Canadian Anaesthetists Society Journal*, 1979, *26*, 492–495.

Edwards, R. M., Tanguay, P., Schwafel, R., Norman, R., Squires, N., & Buchwald, J. Auditory brainstem responses in autistic and control children. Paper presented to the Society for Neurosciences, 1980.

Finitzo-Hieber, T. Auditory brainstem response: Its place in infant audiological evaluations. *Seminars in Speech, Language and Hearing*, 1982, *3* (1), 76–87.

Finitzo-Hieber, T., Simhadri, R., & Hieber, J. P. Abnormalities of the auditory brainstem responses in post-meningitic infants and children. *International Journal of Pediatric Otorhinolaryngology*, 1981, *3*, 275–286.

Fria, T. J. The auditory brainstem response: Background and clinical applications. In D. M. Schwartz & F. H. Bess (Eds.), *Monographs in Contemporary Audiology*, 1980, *2* (2), 1–38.

Frumkin, B., & Rapin, I. Perception of vowels and consonant-vowels of varying duration in language impaired children. *Neuropsychologia*, 1980, *18*, 443–454.

Galambos, R., & Despland, P. A. The auditory brainstem response (ABR) evaluates risk factors for hearing loss in the newborn. *Pediatric Research*, 1980, *14* (2), 159–163.

Galambos, R., & Hecox, K. Clinical applications of the auditory brainstem response. *Otolaryngologic Clinics of North America*, 1978, *11* (3), 709–721.

Galambos, R., Makeig, S., & Talmachoff, P. J. A 40-Hz auditory potential recorded from the human scalp. *Proceedings of the National Academy of Sciences of the United States of America*, 1981, *78* (4), 2643-2647.

Hecox, K., Cone, B., & Blaw, M. E. Brainstem auditory evoked response in the diagnosis of pediatric neurologic disease. *Neurology*, 1981, *31* (7), 832-840.

Hecox, K., & Galambos, R. Brainstem auditory responses in human infants and adults. *Archives of Otolaryngology*, 1974, *99*, 30-33.

Jerger, J. (Ed.). *Modern developments in audiology*. New York: Academic Press, 1973.

Jerger, J. F., & Hayes, D. The cross-check principle in pediatric audiometry. *Archives of Otolaryngology*, 1976, *102*, 614-620.

Jerger, J., Hayes, D., & Jordan, C. Clinical experience with auditory brainstem response audiometry in pediatric assessment. *Ear and Hearing*, 1980, *1* (1), 19-25.

Jerger, J., & Mauldin, L. Prediction of sensorineural hearing level from the brainstem evoked response. *Archives of Otolaryngology*, 1978, *104*, 456-461.

Jerger, J., Neely, J. G., & Jerger, S. Speech, impedance and auditory brainstem response audiometry in brainstem tumors: Importance of a multiple-test strategy. *Archives of Otolaryngology*, 1980, *106* (4), 218-223.

Jewett, D. L., & Williston, J. S. Auditory-evoked far fields averaged from the scalp of humans. *Brain*, 1971, *94*, 681-696.

Kaga, K., Kitazumi, E., & Kodama, K. Auditory brainstem responses of kernicterus infants. *International Journal of Pediatric Otorhinolaryngology*, 1979, *1*, 255-264.

Kileny, P. Auditory brainstem responses as indicators of hearing aid performance. *Annals of Otology*, 1982, *91*, 61-64.

Kileny, P., Connelly, C., & Robertson, C. Auditory brainstem responses in perinatal asphyxia. *International Journal of Pediatric Otorhinolaryngology*, 1980, *2* (2), 147-159.

Kotagal, S., Rosenberg, C., Rudd, D., Dunkle, L. M., & Horenstein, S. Auditory evoked potentials in bacterial meningitis. *Archives of Neurology*, 1981, *38*, 693-695.

Marshall, R. E., Reichert, T. J., Kerley, S. M., & Davis, H. F. Auditory function in newborn intensive care unit patients revealed by auditory brain-stem potentials. *The Journal of Pediatrics*, 1980, *96* (4), 731-735.

Mendel, M. I. Middle evoked potentials in the diagnosis of hearing loss in infants. In S. E. Gerger & G. T. Mencher (Eds.), *Early diagnosis of hearing loss*. New York: Grune & Stratton, 1978, 259-277.

Mendel, M. I., & Goldstein, R. Stability of the early components of the averaged electroencephalic response. *Journal of Speech and Hearing Research*, 1969, *12*, 351-361. (a)

Mendel, M. I., & Goldstein, R. The effect of test conditions on the early components of the averaged electroencephalic response. *Journal of Speech and Hearing Research*, 1969, *12*, 344. (b)

Mendel, M. I., & Goldstein, R. Early components of the averaged electroencephalic response to constant level clicks during all night sleep. *Journal of Speech and Hearing Research*, 1971, *14*, 829-840.

Mjoen, S. ABR in pediatric audiology. Scandinavian symposium on brainstem response (ABR). In T. Lundborg (Ed.). *Scandinavian Audiology Supplement*, 1981, *13*, 141-146.

Mokotoff, B., Schulman-Galambos, C., & Galambos, R. Brainstem auditory evoked responses in children. *Archives of Otolaryngology*, 1977, *103*, 38-43.

Naunton, R. F., & Fernandez, C. (Eds.). *Evoked electrical activity in the auditory nervous system*. New York: Academic Press, 1978.

Nylen, O., & Rosenhall, U. Hemophilus influenzae meningitis and hearing. *International Journal of Pediatric Otorhinolaryngology*, 1979, 97-101.

Ornitz, E. M., & Walter, D. O. The effect of sound pressure waveform on human brainstem auditory evoked responses. *Brain Research*, 1975, *92*, 490–498.

Ozdamar, O., Kvaus, N., & Curvy, F. Auditory brain stem and middle latency responses in a patient with cortical deafness. *Electroencephalography Clinical Neurophysiology*, 1982, *53*, 224–230.

Peters, J. F., Beauchaine, K. A., Reiland, J. K., & Worthington, D. W. ABR in the evaluation of the difficult-to-test patient. *Hearing Instruments*, 1981, *32* (2), 12–14.

Peters, J. F., & Worthington, D. W. Auditory brainstem responses (ABR) in children recovering from meningitis: Preliminary data. *Nicolet Potentials*, 1981, *1*, 4–5.

Picton, T. W. The strategy of evoked potential audiometry. In S. E. Gerger & G. T. Mencher (Eds.), *Early diagnosis of hearing loss*, New York: Grune & Stratton, 1978, 279–307.

Picton, T. W., Woods, D. L., & Baribeau-Braun, J. Evoked potential audiometry. *Journal of Otolaryngology*, 1977, *6*, 90–119.

Robinson, K., & Rudge, P. Abnormalities of the auditory evoked potentials in patients with multiple sclerosis. *Brain*, 1977, *100* (1), 19–40.

Rosenhall, U., & Kankkunen, A. Hearing alterations following meningitis 1. Hearing improvement. *Ear and Hearing*, 1980, *1*, 185–190.

Rowe, M. J., III. The brainstem auditory evoked response in neurological disease: A review. *Ear and Hearing*, 1981, *2* (1), 41–55.

Salamy, A., Mendelson, T., Tooley, W. H., & Chaplin, E. R. Contrasts in brainstem function between normal and high-risk infants in early postnatal life. *Early Human Development*, 1980, *4* (2), 179–185. (a)

Salamy, A., Mendelson, T., Tooley, W. H., & Chaplin, E. R. Differential development of brainstem potentials in healthy and high-risk infants. *Science*, 1980, *210* (4469), 553–555. (b)

Sanders, R. A., Duncan, P. G., & McCullough, D. W. Clinical experience with brain stem audiometry performed under general anesthesia. *Journal of Otolaryngology*, 1979, *8*, 24–32.

Satya-Murti, S., Cacace, A., & Hanson, P. Abnormal AEPs in hereditary motor-sensory neuropathy. *Annals of Neurology*, 1979, *5* (5), 445–448.

Schaffer, A. J., & Angell, M. *Diseases of the newborn* (4th ed.). Philadelphia: W. B. Saunders, 1977.

Schulman-Galambos, C., & Galambos, R. Assessment of hearing. In T. M. Field, A. M. Sostek, S. Goldberg, & H. H. Shuman (Eds.). *Infants born at risk*. Jamaica, NY: Spectrum Publications, 1979, 91–119. (a)

Schulman-Galambos, C., & Galambos, R. Brain Stem evoked response audiometry in newborn hearing screening. *Archives of Otolaryngology*, 179, *105*, 86–90.

Schulman-Galambos, C., & Galambos, R. Brainstem auditory-evoked responses in premature infants. *Journal of Speech and Hearing Research*, 1975, *18*, 456–465.

Sharbrough, F. W., Stockard, J. J., & Aronson, A. E. Brainstem auditory evoked responses in spastic dysphonia. *Transactions of the American Neurological Association*, 1978, *103*, 198–201.

Skoff, B. F., Mirsky, A. F., & Turner, D. Prolonged brainstem transmission time in autism. *Psychiatric Research*, 1980, *2*, 157–166.

Sohmer, H., & Feinmesser, M. Cochlear action potentials recorded from the external ear in man. *Annals of Otolaryngology*, 1967, *76*, 427–435.

Sohmer, H., Feinmesser, M., & Szabo, G. Sources of electrocochleographic responses as studied in patients with brain damage. *Electroencephalography and Clinical Neurophysiology*, 1974, *37*, 663–669.

Sohmer, H., & Student, M. Auditory nerve and brainstem evoked responses in normal, autistic, minimal brain dysfunction and psychomotor retarded children. *Electroencephalography and Clinical Neurophysiology*, 1978, *44*, 380–388.

Sohoel, P., Mair, I. W. S., Elverland, H. H., & Laukli, E. BSER-audiometry in difficult-to-test patients. *Acta Otolaryngolica*, 1979, *Suppl. 360*, 56–57.

Squires, N., Aine, C., Buchwald, J., Norman, R., & Galbraith, G. Auditory brain stems response abnormality in severely and profoundly retarded adults. *Electroencephalography and Clinical Neurophysiology*, 1980, *50*, 172–185.

Starr, A., & Achor, J. Auditory brainstem responses in neurological disease. *Archives of Neurology*, 1975, *32*, 761–768.

Starr, A., & Hamilton, A. E. Correlation between confirmed sites of neurological lesions and abnormalities of far-field auditory brainstem responses. *Electroencephalography and Clinical Neurophysiology*, 1976, *41*, 595–608.

Stockard, J. E., Stockard, J. J., Westmoreland, B. F., & Corfits, J. L. Brainstem auditory-evoked responses: Normal variation as a function of stimulus and subject characteristics. *Archives of Neurology*, 1979, *36*, 823–831.

Stockard, J. E., & Westmoreland, B. F. Technical considerations in the recording and interpretation of the brainstem auditory evoked potential for neonatal neurologic diagnosis. *American Journal of EEG Technology*, 1981, *21*, 31–54.

Stockard, J. J., & Rossiter, V. S. Clinical and pathologic correlates of brain stem auditory response abnormalities. *Neurology*, 1977, *27* (4), 316–325.

Stockard, J. J., Stockard, J. E., & Sharbrough, F. W. Detection and localization of occult lesions with brainstem auditory responses. *Mayo Clinic Proceedings*, 1977, *52* (12), 761–769.

Stockard, J. J., Stockard, J. E., & Sharbrough, F. W. Nonpathologic factors influencing brainstem auditory evoked potentials. *American Journal of EEG Technology*, 1978, *18*, 177–209.

Student, M., & Sohmer, H. Evidence from auditory nerve and brainstem evoked responses for an organic brain lesion in children with autistic traits. *Journal of Autism and Childhood Schizophrenia*, 1978, *8*, 13–20.

Tallal, P., & Piercy, M. Defects of nonverbal auditory perception in children with developmental aphasia. *Nature*, 1973, *241*, 468–469. (a)

Tallal, P., & Piercy, M. Developmental aphasia: Impaired rate of nonverbal processing as a function of sensory modality. *Neuropsyhcologia*, 1973, *11*, 389–398. (b)

Tallal, P., & Piercy, M. Developmental aphasia: Rate of auditory processing and selective imnairment of consonant perception. *Neuropsychologia*, 1974, *12* (1), 83–94.

Tallal, P., & Stark, R. E. Speech acoustic-cue discrimination abilities of normally developing and language-impaired children. *Journal of the Acoustical Society of America*, 1981, *69* (2), 568–574.

Vernon, M. Meningitis and deafness: The problem, its physical, audiological, psychological and educational manifestations in deaf children. *Laryngoscope*, 1967, *77*, 1856–1874.

Vivion, M. C. Clinical status of evoked response audiometry. *Laryngoscope*, 1980, *90* (3), 437–447.

Wilson, L. A. Abnormal brain stem auditory response findings in a neo-natal high-risk population. Personal communication, 1982.

Worthington, D. W., & Peters, J. F. Quantifiable hearing and no ABR: Paradox or error? *Ear and Hearing*, 1980, *1* (5), 281–285.

Yoshie, N. Auditory nerve action potential responses to clicks in man. *Laryngoscope*, 1968, *78*, 198–214.

Noel D. Matkin

Wearable Amplification: A Litany of Persisting Problems

Introduction

The selection of suitable hearing aids is a primary goal when developing comprehensive habilitation programs for hearing-impaired children (Davis & Hardick, 1981; Matkin, 1981a; Ross, 1975). Despite wide acceptance, three major problems persist in terms of implementing this basic principle. Until the following problems are resolved, advances in the audiologic habilitation of children with hearing loss will be limited. First, many children who would benefit from wearable amplification apparently are not wearing hearing aids. This problem exists to some extent among all hearing-impaired children, but is especially prevalent at the two extremes of the hearing loss spectrum. According to two major surveys (Karchmer & Kirwin, 1977; Shepard, Gorga, Davis, & Stelmachowicz, 1981), an appalling number of children having mild hearing losses and a substantial number with profound impairments are not using amplification. Second, a personal review of a large number of patient records from a variety of clinics suggests that very little aided testing is undertaken with many young hearing-impaired children. The suitability of a particular hearing aid apparently is determined on the basis of prior experience with similar cases and such minimal audiologic information as an aided speech detection threshold. Neither approach assures that the instrument is providing adequate amplification of the various phonemes embedded in conversational speech. Third, numerous studies have revealed that many children are wearing hearing aids that are in poor condition (Gaeth & Lounsbury, 1966; Porter, 1973; Robinson & Sterling, 1980; Schell, 1976; Zink, 1972). The fact that many instruments being used by children are poorly maintained suggests that systematic monitoring is not routinely undertaken by audiologists, speech-language clinicians, classroom teachers, and parents. Improvements in hearing aid technology, including increased electro-acoustic flexibility, miniaturization of wearable instruments, and improved earmold acoustics will be of limited benefit to many hearing-impaired children until significant changes in service delivery systems are initiated.

Thus, my purpose in the following sections of this chapter is not only to highlight existing problems, but to speculate on the apparent source of such problems that preclude advances in effectively managing many youngsters with hearing loss. Clinical guidelines are then proposed, which, if adopted in practice as well as in theory, would minimize many of the current shortcomings in hearing aid use by hearing-impaired children. Only by increasing use of wearable amplification will delays in language acquisition and deficits in academic achievement be minimized among youngsters with bilateral sensorineural hearing impairments, or with persistent conductive hearing losses that have not responded to competent medical management.

Determining the Need for a Hearing Aid

The data reported by Karchmer and Kirwin (1977) and Shepard et al. (1981) indicate that many children with mild and profound hearing losses are not using wearable amplification, as compared to those with impairments falling into the moderate or severe hearing-loss categories. The similarity of the findings from these two studies is intriguing in that the Shepard et al. survey was completed within the Iowa public school system where many youngsters are mainstreamed, while the Karchmer and Kirwin data were collected through a survey of special education programs across the nation, including a number of residential schools for the deaf.

The Shepard et al. study indicated that approximately 75% of the children with mild bilateral sensorineural hearing impairments were nonusers, while Karchmer and Kirwin reported that 56% of such children in the special education programs surveyed did not use amplification. If these studies are representative, it appears that less than one-half of all children with bilateral sensorineural hearing losses falling in the range of 26 to 45 dB HL are hearing aid users, regardless of educational setting. One implication of this finding is that physicians, audiologists, and educators apparently believe that a mild bilateral hearing loss does not have an adverse impact upon oral language learning and upon academic achievement in the secondary language areas of reading and writing. Yet, a review of relevant language studies by Young and McConnell (1957), Goetzinger (1962), Kodman (1963), Hamilton and Owrid (1974), Watson (1975), Wohlner (1975), and Quigley (1978) highlights that so-called mild hearing impairments do have adverse effects upon oral-language learning and academic achievement. Language delays of one to two years were not uncommon among samples of children with mild impairments.

Apparently, guidelines developed for adult cases as to the relationship between degree of hearing loss and need for amplification such as reported by Hodgson (1981) are widely used when considering whether or not a child is a candidate for use of a hearing aid. Recall that these guides indicate that when the average hearing loss falls in the mild degree category, amplification will be needed only for special occasions. While such a guideline may be satisfactory when selecting adult patients with intact language skills who may benefit from wearable amplification, it can be argued that the same guideline is quite inappropriate when managing pediatric cases who manifest language delays. Specifically, "special occasion" for a young child with a hearing loss should be viewed as every waking hour during the preschool language-learning years, as well as in subsequent school years. New vocabulary and concepts are being introduced on a daily basis, not only through classroom instruction, but during many home and community activities. Thus, full-time use should be the habilitative goal regardless of the child's age.

In short, the decision as to whether or not a child will benefit from hearing aid use should be based not only upon a review of the audiologic findings, but also upon consideration of the degree to which the child's language development is delayed. In other words, a decision regarding hearing aid use should be a joint professional endeavor during which audiologic findings, language evaluation results, and academic achievement scores are reviewed.

The relationship between language development and achievement in the classroom in terms of concept development, reading, writing, and spelling often is poorly understood. In my clinical experience, many parents express a willingness to proceed with a hearing aid fitting once they understand that use of amplification may not only accelerate the development of receptive and expressive communication skills, but also may minimize academic difficulties. The pervasive effects of a bilateral hearing loss merit careful discussion, not only with parents, but also with the managing physician from whom many parents seek a second opinion about the need for a hearing aid.

Two additional factors appear to account for the reticence of some audiologists to recommend hearing aids for children with mild bilateral impairments. First, preferential seating in the classroom apparently is viewed as a viable alternative to hearing aid use for children with mild losses. However, many classrooms are no longer tightly structured into the traditional lecture format which existed in past decades. Instead, children often are grouped into activity areas with the teacher moving between groups. In such educational settings, the feasibility of the teacher keeping the hearing-impaired child at a close distance to assure maximal auditory input supplemented with visual clues must be seriously questioned. As noted by Sarff (1981), whether a student actually receives preferential seating depends upon a number of variables including the teacher's receptivity to being instructed by an outsider as to the preferred organization of the classroom.

Another factor which apparently deters some audiologists from recommending hearing aid use is the fear that the introduction of wearable amplification may result in either temporary or permanent threshold shifts in mild hearing loss cases. While additional hearing loss related to hearing aid use has been reported by Kinney (1961), Macrae and Farrant (1965), Ross and Lerman (1967), and Macrae (1968), the phenomenon does not appear to be a common one (Reilly, Owens, Uken, McClathehie, & Clarke, 1981). In fact, other investigators question whether hearing aid trauma exists (Barr & Wedenberg, 1965; Bellefleur & Van Dyke, 1968; Madell & Asp, 1970; Markides, 1976; Naunton, 1957). In any case, the probability of further damaging a child's sensorineural auditory mechanism can be substantially minimized by first limiting the maximum output of the hearing aid and then by ongoing monitoring of auditory status. To deny many children the benefits of amplification in an effort to protect the hearing sensitivity of an occasional youngster is a clinical strategy which has little supportive scientific evidence. This issue will be discussed later in this chapter when variables related to the clinical selection of hearing aids are considered.

In the case of children with profound bilateral hearing impairments, the factors which account for nonuse are equally complex and interrelated. Undoubtedly, the amount of benefit offered through amplification is limited when the function of the youngster's auditory system is severely limited by a profound hearing loss. This is particularly true if the level of expectation from hearing aid use is auditory recognition rather than detection of speech (Erber & Witt, 1977). However, it appears that a number of children with profound impairments are initially fitted with hearing aids but do not continue to wear such instruments over time. Perhaps parents as well as teachers become disillusioned as to the benefits of wearable amplification unless a realistic level of expectation is developed initially. Despite limitations, there is evidence that amplified sound can provide substantial prosodic information, as well as improved perception of manner of articulation and the speaker's emotional intent, even when individual words or sentences are not intelligible (Ross, Duffy, Cooker, & Sergeant, 1973). Such benefits may not accrue, however, unless the instrument is provided at an early age and appropriate auditory training is initiated (Ling, Leckie, Pollack, Simser, & Smith, 1981).

It is interesting that the Karchmer and Kirwin study revealed a significantly higher number of nonusers (23%) among children in residential schools, as compared to children with profound hearing losses in the public schools, where Shephard et al. reports a nonuse rate of approximately 15%. One may speculate that many of the nonusers in residental schools are the children of deaf parents, and, further, that they may have one or more deaf teachers. Many such deaf adults, both parents and teachers, often were not exposed to amplification until school age and subsequently found that body aids from several decades ago were of limited benefit. Thus, some deaf children receive minimal, if any, encouragement within the deaf community to continue hearing aid use.

Finally, clinicians need to be aware of other variables which have been identified as characteristic of nonusers. Such pediatric cases can then be more carefully monitored with preventive guidance and counseling initiated before the child abandons hearing aid use. According to Karchmer and Kirwin (1977), educational placement, socioeconomic status, sex, age, and minority status are all factors related to hearing aid use.

In my opinion, the number of children with profound bilateral hearing losses who do not use hearing aids could be reduced if amplification was introduced at an early age and auditory teaching was implemented immediately. Parents and teachers should understand at the outset that while hearing aid use will provide important supplementary information to visual communication—be it oral or total communication—most youngsters with profound hearing impairments do not develop functional speech perception abilities. Through a candid discussion of the advantages and limitations of hearing aid use, disappointment and disillusionment can be minimized. Finally, when there is a high probability that the aid will not be used, it is recommended that appropriate counseling and guidance be initiated as soon as possible.

Selection of an Appropriate Hearing Aid

As with adults, the audiologists must consider four major factors during the clinical selection of hearing aids for children. Specifically, each of the following variables merits careful consideration: the amount of gain needed across frequency to assure audibility of the full acoustic spectrum of speech; the type of hearing aid (ear-level or body); appropriate SSPL 90 or maximum power output to prevent either temporary or permanent threshold shifts; and the preferred arrangement (monaural, binaural, CROS, etc.). These considerations dictate which instruments are selected for trial during the clinical evaluation of a child's aided performance. Each takes on increased importance when one considers the relatively short attention span of many preschoolers during clinical testing, as well as their inability to verbalize quality judgments.

Acoustic Gain

As stated at the outset of this chapter, provision of optimal amplification is an essential feature of an audiologic habilitation program. In other words, identifying a hearing aid, which to the maximum possible extent makes the various acoustic components of a speech message audible, is a primary goal. Unfortunately, several clinical procedures currently used to select a hearing aid do not assure that this goal is achieved.

It has been my observation that the suitabilitiy of a particular hearing aid may be determined by considering *only* the child's aided speech awareness or detection threshold. While the brevity and simplicity of this procedure is appealing when assessing the aided performance of young children, the results can be quite misleading. For example, obtaining an aided speech awareness threshold of 20 to 25 dB HL for two aids may lead an audiologist to assume that the instruments are equally suitable for the child. Yet, as Figure 5-1 demonstrates, aided testing across the various frequencies highlights that with Aid A the critical elements of speech are audible. In contrast, Aid B is adequately amplifying only the lower frequency components of speech, primarily F_1 of vowels, voicing, and nasality cues. In short, Aid A is quite suitable, while Aid B is unsatisfactory. Yet, both aids would have been considered as equivalent in performance if only the aided speech awareness thresholds were compared. Ideally, an aided audiogram will be acquired at the earliest feasible time. With a battery of operant-conditioning techniques, including visual reinforcement audiometry, tangible reinforcement audiometry, and conditioned play audiometry, an aided, as well as an unaided, audiogram can be obtained in most cases before age 1.

Another clinical approach, which has been suggested by Lybarger for selecting a hearing aid, is to choose an instrument with acoustic gain approximately half of the average hearing loss (Berger, Hagberg, & Rane, 1980; Lybarger, 1963). The major shortcomings of the approach are twofold when the goal is to assure audibility of the various acoustic components

FIGURE 5-1
Aided Audiogram for Two Hearing Aids (Aid A = □ Aid B = O),
Which Yielded Speech Awareness Thresholds of 20-25dB HL

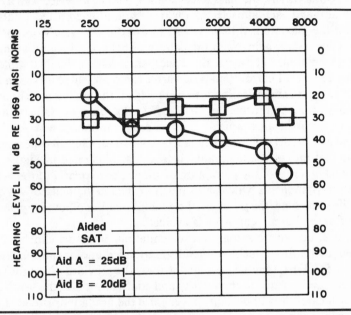

of speech, while avoiding overamplification of low-frequency ambient noise. First, in the case of a mild hearing loss (26-45 dB), there is a good probability of overamplifying the low frequencies, which may result not only in discomfort, but also in upward spread of masking and decrement in speech discrimination (Sweetow, 1977). In contrast, there is the possibility with the "half-gain" approach that a child having a severe hearing loss (66-85 dB) will not be provided with sufficient amplification to detect and recognize the high frequency elements of speech. For example, if an instrument with only 40 dB of gain is used in the presence of an 80 dB impairment, the high frequency voiceless consonants will not be audible during normal conversational speech. For these reasons, the suitability of using this approach with children must be seriously questioned.

Finally, fitting a hearing aid after considering only the 2-cm^3 coupler measurement of an instrument's response cannot be recommended when working with children. As reported by Jirsa (1978), aided thresholds are often better than anticipated due to the small volume of a child's external auditory canal. Further, earmold acoustics can substantially modify aided performance.

In view of the major shortcomings of the preceding approaches, it appears that there is no adequate substitute for an aided sound field audiogram. Ideally, the child under study should be provided with a custom earmold, and each aid selected for trial should be adjusted 10 dB or so below the maximum volume setting to avoid excessive distortion and to allow for reserve gain. With the battery of behavioral-conditioning techniques mentioned above, an aided audiogram can be obtained while using either calibrated narrow bands or warble tones presented in a sound field.

If adequate amplification is to be provided, the audiologist should first establish what consititutes an idealized aided audiogram. Otherwise, there is no reference against which a child's aided performance with a particular brand and model of instrument can be compared. Clinical experience suggests that an aided audiogram, such as that illustrated in Figure 5-2, is optimal in terms of the perception of speech, particularly of the high frequency components which carry much of the intelligibility of a message. At the same time, the problem of overamplification of low-frequency ambient or environmental noise is avoided.

It is important to recognize two limitations in actual clinical practice when attempting to achieve the idealized aided audiogram illustrated in Figure 5-2. First, optimal gain cannot always be provided across the various test frequencies, due to the severity and configuration of the hearing loss. In such cases, it is important to recognize the limitations of aided listening, which can easily be demonstrated by superimposing the speech spectrum upon the audiogram (Nerbonne & Schow, 1980; Olsen & Matkin, 1979). Having a transparency of this information available as an audiogram overlay is a useful clinical tool. Parents can then be counseled as to realistic levels of expectation in terms of their child's anticipated response to amplification. Further, teachers and clinicians can set appropriate habilitation goals by determining the need for supplemental visual input (speechreading or fingerspelling/signing) to supply cues which are missing in the amplified speech message. A second limitation which must also be acknowledged is that the provision of optimal acoustic information to a hearing-impaired child does not assure that even with adequate auditory training and teaching, the youngster will develop the ability to auditorily discriminate all speech signals. In other words, we cannot assume in all cases that the impaired sensorineural mechanism has maintained sufficient integrity to assure a high level of auditory discrimination. Nevertheless, it is apparent that a child cannot develop optimal auditory discrimination if he or she is not provided with audible speech cues.

Fortunately, a major advance in recent years with respect to wearable amplification is that most aids provide a good deal more acoustic flexibility than older units. In other words, it is often possible to suppress an

FIGURE 5-2
Optimal aided audiogram for children as indicated by ■. The approximate boundaries for the spectrum of conversational speech are indicated with the vowel format areas, F1–3, highlighted.

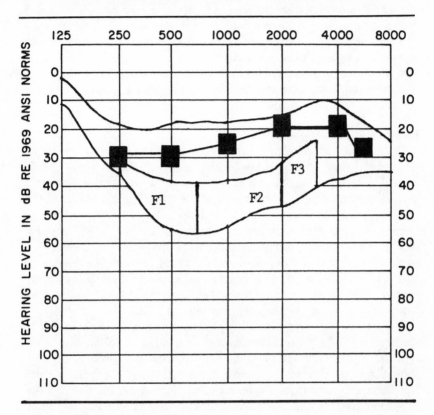

aid's low-frequency response to prevent overamplification in the region of 250 and 500 Hz. At the same time, with improved hearing aid receivers, many contemporary hearing aids provide extended high frequency amplification where many of the voiceless speech sounds occur. In previous years, it was not unnusual for hearing aids to be severely limited in the amount of amplification provided above 3500 Hz. In contrast, many current hearing aids will amplify signals in the frequency region of 3500 to 6000 Hz. A second advance which merits comment is that a substantial body of literature has highlighted the role of earmold acoustics in providing extended high-frequency amplification. By utilizing the so-called horn effect, substantially more gain can be provided in the region of 3000 to 6000 Hz than in previous years. An excellent summary of the effects of earmold acoustics can be found in an article by Killion (1981) and a chapter by Leavitt (1981).

Before concluding this section on the provision of optimal acoustic gain, it is worthwhile to note that there is little evidence that differences in a child's aided discrimination scores can serve as a valid basis for differentiating among various instruments. In many instances, it is not possible to state with assurance whether a depressed discrimination score reflects a poor hearing aid fitting or deficits in either attending behavior or receptive language. Further, there is a lack of research evidence as to what constitutes a significant difference between discrimination scores for most test materials applicable to youngsters.

Hearing Aid Arrangement

Once it has been determined through audiologic and language studies that a child would benefit from hearing aid use, the audiologist should carefully consider whether the fitting should be monaural or binaural. While several authors (Bess & McConnell, 1981; Matkin, 1981b; Ross, 1977) have suggested that hearing-impaired children should be viewed as binaural hearing aid candidates until proven otherwise, there is little evidence that this premise has been put into general clinical practice. For example, Karchmer and Kirwin (1977) reported that of the 151 programs surveyed, only 19.7% of the children were reported as using binaural amplification. In contrast, 40% of the hearing-impaired children in the Iowa public school study were reported as using two instruments (Shepard et al., 1981).

The rationale for recommending binaural hearing aid use is related to the belief that after appropriate auditory training, improved auditory function will be seen in at least two dimensions. First, improved localization should assist the child in quick and accurate location of the speaker, which is a prerequisite to adequate speechreading. Second, binaural-aided hearing should result in improved speech recognition in adverse listening situations, since one aided ear is always favorably placed with respect to the person who is talking. Both of these auditory skills take on additional importance as increasing numbers of hearing-impaired children are mainstreamed into regular classrooms. Many such classrooms have minimal acoustic treatment; thus, children with hearing losses are required to process amplified speech in the presence of background noise and reverberation and, also, to rely heavily upon speechreading to supplement their aided auditory input. As noted by Ross (1977), further research with children is still needed to highlight the benefits of binaural as compared to monaural amplification. In light of the potential benefits of a binaural fitting, however, it behooves the audiologist to assume that the use of two aids will benefit each hearing-impaired child unless there is evidence to the contrary. The second hearing aid can be provided on a trial basis so multiple observations of the child's behavior can be gathered.

Obviously, there are children whose audiologic findings suggest that a recommendation to purchase two hearing aids *cannot* be justified. First, there are those youngsters with bilateral, but asymmetrical, hearing impairments, for whom one ear is essentially nonfunctional with respect to auditory recognition of speech. Limited auditory discrimination abilities may be related either to the profound degree of the loss in the poorer ear or to marked internal distortion due to sensorineural dysfunction. While such children typically are not considered to be candidates for binaural hearing aid use, an alternate hearing aid arrangement—BICROS—may provide additional auditory input as compared to a standard monaural fitting. Second, the potential benefits of binaural amplification for children having a profound bilateral impairment, with only a fragmentary or "corner" audiogram, has been questioned (Matkin, 1981). Third, there is limited evidence that two body instruments located side-by-side on the chest will provide the same binaural advantages as seen with two ear-level aids. Finally, as noted by Jerger & Lewis (1975), binaural hearing aid use is contraindicated in those cases where the use of amplification results in either temporary or permanent shifts in hearing sensitivity, even though the maximum output of the instruments has been appropriately limited.

Unfortunately, it is not possible to determine from any of the published studies the percentage of monaural hearing aid users who would be potential binaural candidates. For this reason, the findings from a large local school system were analyzed while preparing this chapter.

Forty hearing-impaired children of elementary-school age were identified as hearing aid users. Thirty-nine of the youngsters use air-conduction behind-the-ear instruments, while one child with bilateral atresia uses a body aid terminated with a bone-conduction vibrator. Of the 39 children who use ear-level aids, an analysis of the audiologic records suggest that eight youngsters, or 20%, would not be binaural candidates, due to either the degree of loss or extremely limited auditory discrimination in one ear.[1] Of the remaining 31 cases, 12, or 38%, have binaural fittings (a percentage quite similar to that reported in the Iowa study), while 19 are monaural hearing aid users. In other words, 62% of the 31 children who *could* be using two aids, are not. It is of interest that all of these children are mainstreamed into regular classrooms that have little, if any, acoustic treatment; yet they are not provided with either supplemental RF amplification systems or binaural hearing aids as an attempt to minimize the adverse effects of reverberation or noise in the educational environment.

There is a need for systematic clinical investigation to determine the reasons that account for the large number of children who audiologically appear to be candidates for binaural amplification, but who are fitted monaurally. While one may speculate about the contributing factors, the situation will not change until they are better understood.

One clinical strategy that has been found to work well with those children who are being considered for binaural amplification is to initiate hearing aid use with a monaural fitting. Typically, in those cases with a symmetrical impairment, two custom earmolds are procured, and hearing aid use initially is alternated between ears. As soon as it is apparent that both the child *and the parents* have made a satisfactory adjustment to use of one aid, a second aid is introduced for a trial period, unless a difference in aided performance is observed between ears. During the first month that two instruments are being worn, the parents are encouraged to keep a diary relative to key observations or changes in their child's aided performance. At the same time, the child's teacher or clinician is asked to record independent observations of auditory behavior. These notes serve as a basis for discussion between the audiologist and parents when the final decision regarding purchase of a second aid is made.

There is one surprising outcome of this approach that is sometimes encountered. An occasional parent, while positive about his or her child's function with a binaural fitting, elects not to proceed with the use of two instruments. This reluctance is related to the perception that the child appears more handicapped when two aids are used.

Type of Hearing Aid

One of the most apparent changes in the area of wearable amplification is the increasing number of behind-the-ear instruments being worn, not only by adults, but by young children, including toddlers. In 1979, ear-level instruments represented 97% of all hearing aid sales in the United States, while body aids represented only 3% (Bess & McConnell, 1981). Recall that a decade or so ago, body aids were routinely recommended for most children, since they were considered to offer greater electroacoustic flexibility, higher acoustic gain, and better durability. Many contemporary postauricular instruments provide acoustic gain approaching that of body aids. Further, variable tone and power output controls often are standard features.

A recent study of hearing aid users revealed that approximately 72% of the children surveyed in the province of British Columbia wear postauricular aids (Clarke & Rogers, 1979). In contrast, 39 of 40 (97.5%) elementary-aged youngsters in the Tucson Unified School District now use behind-the-ear instruments, while 17 of 27 youngsters (63%) in the local preschool center for hearing-impaired children wear postauricular aids. Of the 10 children who do wear body instruments, 6 have profound impairment, while the remaining 4 are either infants or toddlers.

The two most frequently cited advantages of ear-level aids are the provision of a full binaural advantage, available since the instruments' microphones are located at each ear, and the elimination of clothing noise. In addition, there is no reported evidence of greater repair problems. In fact, some common problems encountered with body aids, including food in microphones and broken cords, are eliminated. Finally, ear-level instruments are more cosmetically appealing to some parents and older children. Comfort may also be a factor leading to more consistent use.

At present, body type aids typically are reserved for use with:

1. Children having profound impairments where better aided responses are obtained with body, rather than powerful ear-level, instruments;

2. Infants and toddlers whose small pinnas do not provide sufficient stability to keep postauricular aids in place;

3. Children with congenital atresia requiring the use of bone-conduction amplification;

4. Children, usually with severe or profound impairments, for whom it is not possible to obtain an earmold fit that precludes feedback as a constant problem;

5. Older children with major motor deficits and limited manual dexterity, but who should be encouraged to develop independent skills in hearing aid use and care.

While all in-the-ear and eyeglass instruments account for 27% of all retail hearing aid sales, these instruments are rarely used with young children. However, such aids are preferred and successfully used by some hearing-impaired teenagers.

While numerous parents and clinicians appear increasingly enthusiastic about fitting young children with ear-level aids, a word of caution is needed. Eight of 11 preschoolers with severe and profound losses recently evaluated were found to be receiving limited benefit from such aids, because parents had set the instruments to a reduced volume setting to avoid constant feedback problems. As reported by Clark, Watkins, Reese, Allen, Olsen, and Berg (1975), youngsters under age 3, on the average, require new earmolds every 2 to 3 months to assure an adequate seal. In short, elimination of the feedback problem requires constant monitoring by parents when ear-level instruments are used with young children. There also is considerable expense involved in procuring new earmolds, especially in those instances where two aids are used.

In contrast to a previously restricted view of hearing aids for children, the prevailing premise now appears to be that any hearing aid arrangement successfully utilized with adults should be considered for use with children. In addition to conventional monaural and binaural ear-level fittings, success in using CROS and BICROS-type instruments with children has been reported by Matkin and Thomas (1972), Maering and Brunt (1975), Shapiro (1977), and Clarke & Rogers (1979).

Limiting Maximum Output

Caution must be exercised when adjusting the SSPL 90 of hearing aids selected for use with children. While neither temporary nor permanent threshold shifts from hearing aid use appear to be a common phenomena, there is evidence that the utilization of wearable amplification can be traumatic in selected cases (Heffernan & Simons, 1979; Jerger & Lewis, 1975; Reilly et al., 1980). Thus, the possibility of hearing aids causing further hearing loss cannot be dismissed. An analysis of audiologic data collected for 253 children with bilateral sensorineural impairment, who used hearing aids, revealed that the prevalance of so-called hearing aid trauma was approximately 1 in 80 (Matkin, 1973). At that time, the average maximum output of the instruments was restricted to 130 dB SPL, regardless of the degree of hearing loss.

Rintlemann and Bess (1977), after reviewing the major publications relating potential hearing loss and amplification, recommended that instruments with saturation outputs approaching 130 dB SPL should be used with extreme caution, and then only with children having severe or profound losses. An SSPL of 120 dB was viewed as the maximum acceptable output for those youngsters with mild and moderate impairments.

At present, there is increasing clinical evidence that the hazards to residual hearing due to overamplification can be markedly reduced by determining the maximum SSPL 90, after considering the degree of hearing loss. For the past three years, the following guidelines have been used in the University of Arizona Hearing Clinics: an output of 125 dB SPL is the maximum used, and only with those children having profound impairments. In contrast, 120 dB SPL is used with youngsters having moderate to severe impairments, while 115 dB SPL is the maximum output recommended for those with mild losses. It should be kept in mind, however, that the real ear output may exceed these values, due to the small volume of the external auditory canal in children as compared to a 2-cm^3 coupler. Since adopting the preceding guidelines, the question of hearing aid trauma has been raised in only one case.

Since there is no reliable objective technique for determining a child's loudness-discomfort level, careful observation of the child's response behaviors to loud sounds should be made. Further, reduction of the SSPL 90 may be necessary if adverse reactions to intense stimuli are noted after the initial period of adjustment to hearing aid use.

Monitoring Hearing Aid Performance

As mentioned in the introduction, the third major and persisting problem relating to hearing aid use by children is that many such instruments are in poor condition. Since this issue was repeatedly highlighted ten years or so ago (Gaeth & Lounsbury, 1966; Porter, 1973; Zink, 1972), one might assume that the habilitative strategies for minimizing the problem would now be widely implemented. Yet, a recent report by Robinson and Sterling (1980) suggests that the situation has not changed to any appreciable extent. Through an electroacoustic analysis of 97 hearing aids, they found that 39 (40%) instruments were not functioning within the manufacturer's specifications.

Equally discouraging is the analysis of responses on a questionnaire designed to assess parents' knowledge of their child's hearing aid (Blair, Wright, & Pollard, 1981). Specifically, parental understanding of hearing aids was evaluated relative to their response to basic questions about earmolds, batteries, and the benefits of amplification. In a sample of 96 parents, 60% demonstrated little or no knowledge of their child's hearing aid. Robinson and Sterling reported equally discouraging results on the basis of parent interview. For example, 32 of 97 parents were either uncertain or grossly misinformed with respect to the fundamental issue of projected battery life for their child's hearing aid. If these findings are representative of parents at large, then it should not be surprising that as many as half of the instruments used by children are poorly maintained or improperly worn.

The basis for this problem appears to be multifaceted and related to one or more flaws in service-delivery systems. For example, discussion during a recent conference of amplification revealed that responsibility for parent education and guidance is readily shifted among professionals. One typical example of relegating responsibility is that the audiologist recommending the aid assumed that the hearing aid dispenser would orient the parents to hearing aid function and care, while the dispenser assumed the child's classroom teacher would assume this responsibility. As a result, the parents did not receive adequate instruction relative to hearing aid monitoring and maintenance by anyone. Further, a national study by Rawlings and Trybus (1978) revealed that only 29% of the educational programs surveyed have daily hearing aid checks, while 19% reported that the function of hearing aids is never evaluated either formally or informally. Yet, a 5-year survey of hearing aids revealed that through daily inspections of the instruments, the average number of malfunctions per child was reduced by approximately 50% (Kemker, McConnell, Logan, & Green, 1979).

A second potential basis of the problem may be related to the phenomenon of "too much, too soon." That is, instruction in hearing aid care may be provided soon after the child's hearing loss is identified, and during a period that many parents are actively dealing with their own grieving process. As a result, they do not process and retain the information, even though it was adequately presented. The problem, as highlighted by Luterman (1979), suggests that hearing aid orientation for parents not only needs to be appropriately timed, but also should be an ongoing process. To assure sufficient redundancy relative to hearing aid orientation, printed materials including trouble-shooting guides should be available as handouts to supplement verbal instruction.

Finally, Luterman (1979) suggests that the quality of maintenance of a child's hearing aid may subtly, but directly, reflect the parents' acceptance of the youngster's hearing loss. Stated differently, a poor record of hearing aid care may not in some cases be an indication of limited education and guidance, but the parents' reluctance to accept the need for hearing aid use. Clinicians must keep in mind that a hearing impairment is an invisible handicap only until hearing aid use is initiated. Unfortunately, many audiologists have received minimal formal training in counseling and, as a consequence, question their own clinical competence in this area (Flahive & White, 1981).

Given that there is little, if any, evidence of improvement during the past decade, the implementation of the following recommendations is mandatory. First, the audiologist who makes the hearing aid recommendation should assume full responsibility for education and guidance of the parents relative to hearing aid surveillance and maintenance. As a minimum, a printed hearing aid trouble-shooting guide, a battery tester, and a hearing aid stethoscope should be available in the home, with assurance that the parents have the skills and commitment to make daily hearing aid checks. Ideally, the child's teacher will provide reinforcement and encouragement relative to this basic, yet critical, parental responsibility. Second, the audiologist must be sensitive to each parent's level of understanding and educational background, so that such instruction is individualized. Third, such verbal instruction should be supplemented with appropriate handouts, pamphlets, and reprints, again as an alternate form of reinforcement. Even preschoolers should be included in hearing aid orientation, so that as they mature they can assume independence in caring for their aids. Finally, hearing aid orientation should be an ongoing endeavor and a key component of service delivery during each return visit to the managing audiologist.

Conclusion

As this chapter is concluded, the importance of consistent and systematic monitoring of hearing-impaired children must be stressed. Many of the persisting problems highlighted in the preceding discussion cannot be minimized unless the managing audiologist maintains ongoing contact with the hearing-impaired child, the parents, and the classroom teacher. Scheduling audiologic re-evaluations every 3 months during the first year after a child is identified as hearing-impaired and fitted with a hearing aid is beneficial.

There are at least four major reasons why 6-month re-evaluations during the remaining preschool years, and then yearly re-evaluations during the school years, should be scheduled. First, the auditory status of each child should be monitored for change. Progressive sensorineural hearing losses of unknown etiology, decrements in hearing sensitivity due to middle ear dysfunction, and threshold shifts from the use of amplification may all be encountered among hearing-impaired youngsters. Such changes require otologic as well as audiologic intervention. Second, assessing the electroacoustic function of the child's hearing aids and monitoring the adequacy of the earmold fit are of prime importance if maximum benefit from the instrument is to be realized. Third, evidence that the auditory component of the education/habilitation program is adequate should be apparent if measures of aided auditory discrimination reveal improved auditory performance over time. Fourth, time should be set aside during each re-evaluation to monitor the parents, both in terms of their acceptance of hearing aid use as well as their ability and ongoing commitment to maintain their child's hearing aids in optimal working condition. Each of these reasons alone serves as sufficient justification to schedule periodic audiologic re-evaluations; collectively, they make ongoing monitoring mandatory.

Note

[1]A similar analysis of the audiologic records of 17 preschoolers suggest that 3 children, or 18%, would not be considered as binaural hearing aid candidates, due to the profound degree of impairment in the poorer ear.

References

Barr, B., & Wedenberg, E. Prognosis of perceptive hearing loss in children with respect to genesis and use of hearing aid. *Acta Otolaryngologica,* 1965, *59,* 462-474.

Bellefleur, P.A., & Van Dyke, R.C. The effects of high gain amplification on children in a residential school for the deaf. *Journal of Speech and Hearing Research,* 1968, *11,* 343-347.

Berger, K.W., Hagberg, E.N., & Rane, R.L. A re-examination of the one-half gain rule. *Ear and Hearing,* 1980, *I,* 223-225.

Bess, F.H., & McConnell, F.E. *Audiology, education, and the hearing impaired child.* St. Louis: C.V. Mosby, 1981.

Blair, J.C., Wright, K., & Pollard, G. Parental knowledge and understanding of hearing loss and hearing aids. *The Volta Review,* 1981, *83,* 375-382.

Clark, T., Watkins, S., Reese, R., Allen, A., Olsen, S., & Berg, F. *Programming for hearing impaired infants through amplification and home intervention.* Logan: Utah State University, 1975.

Clarke, B.R., & Rogers, W.T. The relationship between personal hearing aids and selected characteristics of hearing-impaired students. *Journal of Audiological Research,* 1979, *19,* 23-26.

Davis, J.M., & Hardick, E.J. *Rehabilitative audiology for children and adults.* New York: John Wiley, 1981.

Erber, N.P., & Witt, L.H. Effects of stimulus intensity on speech perception by deaf children. *Journal of Speech and Hearing Disorders,* 1977, *42,* 271-278.

Flahive, M.J., & White, S.C. Audiologists and counseling. *Academy of Rehabilitative Audiology,* 1981, *14,* 274-287.

Gaeth, J.H., & Lounsbury, E. Hearing aids and children in elementary schools. *Journal of Speech and Hearing Disorders,* 1966, *31,* 289-293.

Goetzinger, C.P. Effects of small perceptive losses on language and on speech discrimination. *The Volta Review,* 1962, *64,* 408-414.

Hamilton, P., & Owrid, H.L. Comparison of hearing impairment and sociocultural disadvantage in relation to verbal retardation. *British Journal of Audiology,* 1974, *8,* 27-32.

Heffernan, H.P., & Simons, M.R. Temporary increase in sensorineural hearing loss with hearing aid use. *Annals of Otology,* 1979, *88,* 86-91.

Hodgson, W.R. Clinical measure of hearing performance. In W.R. Hodgson & P.H. Skinner (Eds.), *Hearing aid assessment and use in audiologic habilitation.* Baltimore: Williams & Wilkins, 1981.

Jerger, J.F., & Lewis, N. Binaural hearing aids: Are they dangerous for children? *Archives of Otology.* 1975, *101,* 480-483.

Jirsa, R.E. Relationship of acoustic gain to aided threshold improvement in children. *Journal of Speech and Hearing Disorders,* 1978, *43,* 348-352.

Karchmer, M.A., & Kirwin, L.A. *The use of hearing aids by hearing impaired students in the United States.* Washington, DC: Office of Demographic Studies, Gallaudet College, 1977.

Kemker, F.J., McConnell, F., Logan, S.A., & Green, B.W. A field study of children's hearing aids in a school environment. *Language, Speech, and Hearing Services in Schools,* 1979, *10,* 47-53.

Killion, M. C. Earmold further options for wideband hearing aids. *Journal of Speech and Hearing Disorders,* 1981, *46,* 10-20.

Kinney, C.E. The further destruction of partially deafened children's hearing by the use of powerful hearing aids. *Annals of Otology,* 1961, *70,* 828-835.

Kodman, F. Educational status of hard of hearing children in the classroom. *Journal of Speech and Hearing Disorders,* 1963, *28,* 297-299.

Leavitt, R. Earmolds: Acoustic and structural considerations. In W.R. Hodgson & P.H. Skinner (Eds.), *Hearing aid assessment and use in audiologic habilitation.* Baltimore: Williams & Wilkins, 1981.

Ling, D., Leckie, D., Pollack, D., Simser, J., & Smith, A. Syllable reception by hearing-impaired children trained from infancy in auditory-oral programs. *The Volta Review*, 1981, *83*, 451-457.

Luterman, D. *Counseling parents of hearing-impaired children* Boston: Little, Brown, 1979.

Lybarger, S.F. *Simplified fitting system for hearing aids,* Canonsburg, PA: Radioear Corp., 1963.

Macrae, J.H. Deterioration of the residual hearing of children with sensorineural deafness. *Acta Otolaryngologica,* 1968, *66,* 33-39.

Macrae, J.H., & Farrant, R.H. The effect of hearing aid use on the residual hearing of children with sensorineural deafness. *Annals of Otology,* 1965, *74,* 409-419.

Madell, J.R., & Asp, C.W. The effects of hearing aid amplification on pure tone thresholds of preschool deaf children. Paper presented at the American Speech and Hearing Association Convention, New York, 1977.

Maering, R.J., & Brunt, M.A. Benefit obtained by children from wearing CROS hearing aids, *Journal of Audiological Research,* 1975, *15,* 270-275.

Markides, A. The effect of hearing aid use on the user's residual hearing. *Scandanavian Audiology,* 1976, *5,* 205-210.

Matkin, N.D. Some essential features of a pediatric audiological evaluation. In E. Kampp (Ed.), *Evaluation of hearing handicapped children.* Fifth Danavox Symposium, Ebeltoft, Denmark, 1973.

Matkin, N.D. Amplification for children: Current status and future priorities. In F.H. Bess, B.A. Freeman, & J.S. Sinclair (Eds.), *Amplification in education.* Washington, DC: Alexander Graham Bell Association for the Deaf, 1981. (a)

Matkin, N.D. Hearing aids for children. In W.R. Hodgson & P.H. Skinner (Eds.), *Hearing aid assessment and use in audiologic habilitation.* Baltimore: Williams & Wilkins, 1981. (b)

Matkin, N.D., Thomas, J. The utilization of CROS hearing aids by children. Audiological Library Series #8, Maico Hearing Instruments 10, 1972.

Naunton, R.F. The effect of hearing aid use upon the user's residual hearing. *Laryngoscope,* 1957, *67,* 569-576.

Nerbonne, M.A., & Schow, R.L. Auditory stimuli in communication. In R.L. Schow & M.A. Nerbonne (Eds.), *Introduction to aural rehabilitation.* Baltimore: University Park Press, 1980.

Olsen, W.O., & Matkin, N.D. Speech discrimination. In W.F. Rintelmann (Ed.), *Hearing assessment.* Baltimore: University Park Press, 1979.

Porter, T. Hearing aids in a residential school, *American Annals of the Deaf,* 1973, *118,* 31-33.

Quigley, S.P. Effects of early hearing impairment on normal language development. In F.N. Martin (Ed.), *Pediatric audiology.* Englewood Cliffs, NJ: Prentice-Hall, 1978.

Rawlings, B., & Trybus, R. Personnel, facilities, and services available in schools and classes for hearing impaired children in the United States, *American Annals of the Deaf,* 1978, *123,* 99-114.

Reilly, K., Owens, E., Uken, D., McClathchie, A.D., & Clarke, R. Progressive hearing loss in children: Hearing aids and other factors. *Journal of Speech and Hearing Disorders,* 1981, *46,* 328-334.

Rintelmann, W.F., & Bess, F.H. High level amplification and potential hearing loss in children. In F.H. Bess (Ed.), *Childhood deafness: Causation, assessment, and management.* New York: Grune & Stratton, 1977.

Robinson, D.O., & Sterling, G.R. Hearing aids and children in school: A follow-up study, *The Volta Review,* 1980, *82,* 229-235.

Ross, M. Hearing aid selection for preverbal hearing impaired children. In M. Pollack (Ed.), *Amplification for the hearing impaired.* New York: Grune & Stratton, 1975.

Ross, M. Binaural vs. monaural hearing aids. In F.H. Bess (Ed.), *Childhood deafness: Causation, assessment, and management,* New York: Grune & Stratton, 1977.

Ross, M., Duffy, R.J., Cooker, H.S., & Sergeant, R.J. Contribution of the lower audible frequencies to the recognition of emotions, *American Annals of the Deaf,* 1973, *118,* 37-42.

Ross, M., Lerman, J. Hearing aid usage and its effect upon residual hearing, *Archives of Otolaryngology,* 1967, *86,* 639-644.

Sarff, L.S. An innovative use of free field amplification in regular classrooms. In R. Roser & M. Downs (Eds.), *Auditory disorders in school children.* New York: Thieme-Stratton, 1981.

Schell, Y. Electroacoustic evaluation of hearing aids worn by public school children, *Audiological and Hearing Education,* 1976, *2,* 7-15.

Shapiro, I. Children's use of CROS hearing aids, *Archives of Otolaryngology,* 1977, *103,* 712-716.

Shepard, N.T., Gorga, M.P., Davis, J.M., & Stelmachowicz, P.G. Characteristics of hearing-impaired children in the public schools: Part I—Demographic data. *Journal of Speech and Hearing Disorders,* 1981, *46,* 123-129.

Sweetow, R.W. Temporal and spread of masking effects from extended low frequency amplification. *Journal of Audiological Research,* 1977, *17,* 161-170.

Watson, C.G. A study of short term visual memory skills and relationship to certain aspects of language in selected groups of hearing-impaired children. Unpublished doctoral dissertation, Northwestern University, 1975.

Wohlner, L.R. An investigation of certain verbal and gestural communication abilities in hard-of-hearing and normal hearing children. Unpublished doctoral dissertation, Northwestern University, 1975.

Young, C., & McConnell, F. Retardation of vocabulary development in hard-of-hearing children. *Exceptional Children,* 1957, *33,* 268-270.

Zink, G. Hearing aids children wear: A longitudinal study of performance, *The Volta Review,* 1972, *74,* 41-51.

Supplemental Readings

Avery, C.B. Rehabilitation of the hearing impaired child. *ENT J.,* 1978, *57,* 71-80.

Beggs, W.D., & Foreman, D.L. Sound localization and early binaural experience in the deaf. *British Journal of Audiology,* 1980, *14,* 41-48.

Bench, J., & Cotter, S. Predicting children's use of hearing aids, *Teach Deaf,* 1978, *2,* 159-162.

Bendet, R.M. A public school hearing aid maintenance program, *Volta Review,* 1980, *85,* 149-155.

Bergenstoff, H. On the problem of fitting an individual hearing aid: A case story, *Scandanavian Audiology,* 1979, Suppl. 6, 438-449.

Blair, J.C. Effects of amplification, speech reading, and classroom environments on reception of speech, *Volta Review,* 1977, *79,* 443-449.

Byrne, D. Selection of hearing aids for severely deaf children. *British Journal of Audiology,* 1978, *12,* 9-22.

Clarke, B.R. Children who wear individual hearing aids in British Columbia, Canada, *Scandanavian Audiology,* 1979, *8,* 131-136.

Danhauer, J.L. Professional and lay observers' impressions of preschoolers wearing hearing aids, *Journal of Speech and Hearing Disorders,* 1980, *45,* 415-422.

Fabritius, H.F. Audiological treatment of preschool children with hearing impairments, *Acta Oto-laryngology,* 1976, *82,* 268-270.

Hirsch, I.J. Psychological aspects of early auditory education, *Journal of the Royal Society of Medicine*, 1980, *73*, 611-616.

Larsen, T.G. Auditory stimulation of very young children, *Scandanavian Audiology*, 1980, Suppl. 10, *10*, 105-111.

Ling, D. Hearing aids and the use of residual hearing. *Australian Journal of Human Communication Disorders*, 1976, *4*, 9-14.

Lourensz, C. An audiological approach to classroom practice, *Teach. Deaf*, *2*, 124-129.

Ludvigsen, C. Acoustic aspects of auditory training with and without hearing aid. *Scandanavian Audiology*, 1980, Suppl. 10, 69-83.

Madell, J.R. Amplification for hearing-impaired children: Basic considerations. *Journal of Communication Disorders*, 1978, *11*, 125-135.

Markides, A., Huntington, A., & Kettlety, A. Comparative speech discrimination abilities of hearing-impaired children achieved through infra-red, radio, and conventional hearing aids, *Teach. Deaf*, 1980, *4*, 5-14.

Martin, M.C., Grover, B.C., Worrall, J.J., & Williams, V. The effectiveness of hearing aids in a school population. *British Journal of Audiology*, 1976, *10*, 33-40.

Miller, A.L. Hearing loss and your child, Springfield, IL: Charles C. Thomas, 1980.

O'Connell, C., Bajjalieh, S., & Lee Charlton, J. Research relating to children, ERIC/ECE Bulletin 40, 1978.

O'Loughlin, B.J. Evaluation of a three channel compression amplification system on hearing-impaired children, *Australian Journal of Audiology*, 1980, *2*, 1-9.

Ross, M., & Calvert, D.R. Guidelines for audiology programs in educational settings for hearing-impaired. *Volta Review*, 1977, *79*, 153-161.

Rubin, M. The relation between impedance findings and hearing aid selection for hearing-impaired infants. *Volta Review*, 1979, *81*, 436-440.

Schiff, M., & Cohen, I.J. Selection of hearing aids. *Otolaryngology*, Clinics of North America, 1979, *12*, 677-692.

Schwartz, D.M., & Larson, V.D. A comparison of three hearing aid evaluation procedures for young children. *Archives of Otolaryngology*, 1977, *103*, 401-406.

Spitzer, J.B. Trends in audiologic services to hearing-impaired children, *Volta Review*, 1981, *83*, 150-155.

Walter, G.G. The effect of prolonged hearing aid use on the communication skills of young deaf adults, *American Annals of the Deaf*, 1978, *123*, 548-554.

Wilbur, L. Amplification for the adolescent, *Volta Review*, 1978, *80*, 296-300.

Fred H. Bess
Susan A. Logan

Amplification in the Educational Setting

Introduction

It is generally agreed that appropriate amplification is an essential component in the successful management of hearing-impaired children. Amplification represents the primary means for the hearing-impaired child to receive the acoustic information so important for language development and learning. In view of the acknowledged importance of amplification for the hearing impaired, it is surprising to find that in actual practice there is a lack of appreciation on the part of both audiologists and educators with regard to the rehabilitative value of these prosthetic devices. There are numerous examples of the audiologist's and educator's failure to appreciate the benefits children realize from hearing aids. More than one-half of the hearing aids worn by children in the United States are found to be in poor working order. In addition, many local educational agencies fail to employ programs designed to monitor and maintain children's hearing aids. Finally, graduate-training programs continue to provide students with only limited exposure to the use and care of various amplification systems commonly employed in the educational setting.

This chapter is written in recognition of the importance of amplification for children in the educational setting. The chapter focuses on several areas including the acoustic environment, the types of hearing aid systems used in education, the selection and evaluation of educational systems, and the status of amplification in education.

The Acoustic Climate

An important consideration for amplification in education is the acoustical environment encountered by hearing-impaired children. It is recognized, for example, that high noise levels and prolonged reverberation can adversely affect the signal-to-noise ratio (S/N) reaching the child's ear. Furthermore, hearing-impaired listeners are known to exhibit greater difficulty understanding speech than normal hearers under the same noise conditions. This section offers a review of some of the more salient areas associated with the acoustic climate.

Noise Levels in the Learning Environment

The accepted definition of noise is "any unwanted sound" (Glorig, 1958, p.3). Children are exposed to a variety of "unwanted sounds" in their daily activities. Typical noise environments encountered by children include the home, classrooms, auditorium/theaters, churches, gymnasiums, stores and restaurants. Unfortunately, the noise levels generated in many of these indoor activities far exceed acceptable values for hearing-impaired children. According to Fourcin, Joy, Kennedy, et al. (1980), traditional classrooms for the hearing impaired should not exceed 30 to 35 dB(A) and classrooms for activity areas (i.e., arts, crafts) should not exceed 45 dB(A). Yet, seldom if ever, does a classroom or activity area meet such specifications. As early as 1965, Sanders demonstrated that the average noise levels measured in occupied classrooms ranged from 52 dB(B) to 69 dB(B), depending on the type of classroom. Interestingly, there was a trend toward higher noise levels for the lower grade classrooms. More recent data on noise levels in the classroom indicate that conditions have not improved since the initial study by Sanders. Figure 6-1 represents typical noise levels obtained in 19 modern classrooms used by hearing-impaired children and youth. This figure presents the medians and ranges of the overall noise levels for both unoccupied and occupied conditions. It is seen that in the unoccupied condition, the median noise level was 41 dB on the A rating scale and 58 dB on the C rating scale. When occupied, however, the median noise levels increased by 15 dB on the A scale and 5 dB on the C scale. Some of the various factors thought to be contributing to high noise levels were absence of sound-treated materials to the furniture and reflective surfaces of the room. The high noise levels measured in these current-day classrooms suggest a need to place greater emphasis on the acoustic treatment of classrooms for the hearing impaired.

As noted earlier, high noise levels measured in these various rooms adversely affect S/N ratios reaching the children's ears. The S/N ratio is thought to be the most important consideration for speech understanding.

FIGURE 6-1
Medians and Ranges of the Overall Noise Levels of 19 Classrooms for Both Unoccupied and Occupied Conditions.

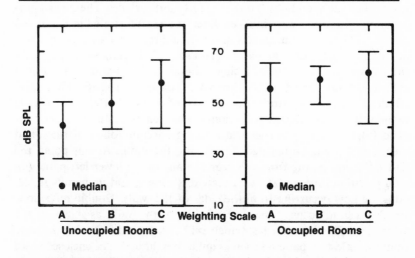

The level of a teacher's voice, measured at one meter from the source, ranges from 67 to 78 dB and, at 7 meters, the intensity ranges from 57 to 62 dB (Pearsons, Bennett, & Fidell, 1977). Although normal-hearing children may operate efficiently under such conditions, Gengel (1971) has suggested that S/N ratios of +15 to +20 dB, or more, are necessary for the hearing-impaired listener to function in a noise-filled environment. More specifically, a S/N ratio of 33 dB is needed for the identification of consonants, and 22 dB is necessary for vowel identification (Gengel, 1971; Ross, Brackett, & Maxon, 1982). Actual kindergarten and elementary classroom S/N ratios have been reported to range from -6 dB to +6 dB (Bess & McConnell, 1981; Sanders, 1965). In other functional activity areas such as churches, restaurants, stores, and gymnasiums, where the noise levels are presumably higher than in classrooms, the S/N ratios would be even less favorable.

Another factor that affects the S/N ratio is the distance between the sound source and the listener. The intensity of a sound decreases inversely with the square of the distance from the sound source. Hence, speech intensity decreases by 6 dB as the distance between the talker and the listener is doubled. The problems created by distance are recognized as the primary disadvantage of the personal hearing aid.

Reverberation

High noise levels are not the only factors that lead to listening difficulties for hearing-impaired children. Reverberation is also an important consideration. Reverberation is defined as the persistence of sound within an enclosed space when the sound waves reflect off of hard surfaces. The typical propagation of a sound wave in an enclosed room is illustrated in Figure 6-2 (Sabine, 1957). The four panels in this figure represent a horizontal section of a typical classroom having plain sound-reflecting walls. The solid circle represents the front of a single sound wave, while the dotted lines indicate the directions in which the sound is traveling. The upper left panel (a) illustrates the wave front at only 1/200 of a second after it has left the sound source. Note that no reflections have taken place. In the upper right panel (b), the wave front is now at 1/100 of a second following the sound source, and it has propagated further into the room. At this point, the first reflection occurs from the nearest wall. In the lower left panel (c), a propagation time of 1/50 of a second is shown, and numerous reflections are now occurring from the sides of the walls. Double reflections are also seen to occur at the end and sides of the walls, as shown by the dotted line. Finally, in the last panel, 1/17 of a second following the wave front the reflection pattern becomes quite complicated. The enclosed space is literally filled with sound waves, all traveling in different directions throughout the room. Generally speaking, there are two effects that can occur as a consequence of this multiple reflection affect (Sabine, 1957). First, there is an increase in the sound pressure that is caused by the reflections. If a continuous sound is made, the listener in the room will receive not only the direct sound waves, but the reflected waves as well. Hence, the combined sound pressure level of the direct and the reflected sound waves will be greater than that of the direct sound wave alone. The second basic effect of a multiple reflection is the actual reverberation itself. The harder the surfaces within the enclosed space, the longer the sound waves will continue to persist in the classroom.

With the possible exception of an anechoic chamber, all rooms exhibit some degree of reverberation. The reverberation time is generally described as the amount of time for sound to decrease by 60 dB, following termination of the signal. The human ear can integrate repetitive sounds that arrive up to .08 seconds after the original sound wave has been terminated. In fact, some investigators have suggested that the waves reflected at an interval .02 to .03 seconds actually enhance the speech understanding of normal hearers (Olsen, 1981). Unfortunately, however, such is not the case for the hearing impaired listener. In general, it is not unusual for classrooms to exhibit reverberation times ranging from .02 to an excess of 1.0 seconds (Bess & McConnell, 1981; Olsen, 1977, 1981).

FIGURE 6-2
Propagation of a Sound Wave in an Enclosed Room (horizontal section) (Redrawn from H. J. Sabine. Acoustical Materials. In C. M. Harris, (Ed.), *Handbook of Noise Control*. New York: McGraw-Hill, 1957.)

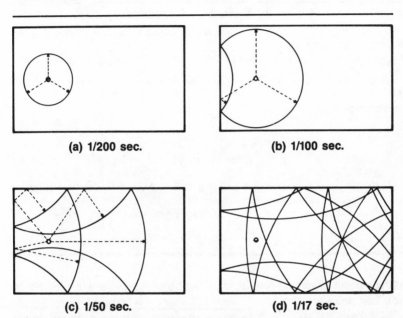

(a) 1/200 sec.   (b) 1/100 sec.

(c) 1/50 sec.   (d) 1/17 sec.

Note: Solid circle represents the front of sound wave and dotted lines denote the direction of the wave.

Effects of Noise and Reverberation on Speech Recognition

It has already been noted that both noise and reverberation can adversely affect one's ability to understand speech. In fact, studies on the effects of noise and reverberation on speech recognition in the hearing impaired suggest that the two factors are not simply additive, but perhaps even synergistic. That is, the combination of noise and increased reverberation time can be more deleterious to speech recognition in the hearing impaired than one would predict by the simple addition of the effects of both (Bess & Gravel, 1981). An example of the combined effects of reverberation time and noise on word recognition for a group of hearing-impaired children is seen in Table 6-1. These data represent the mean word recognition scores for a group of hearing-impaired children who are wearing amplification

Table 6-1
Mean Word Recognition Scores for a Group of Hearing-Impaired Children With Hearing Aids Under Various Noise and Reverberant Conditions

Reverberation time (seconds)	Signal-to-Noise ratio (dB)			
	Quiet	+12	+6	0
0.0 (nonreverberant)	83	70	60	39
0.4	74	60	52	28
1.2	45	41	27	11

NOTE: Adapted from T. Finitzo-Hieber & T. W. Tillman. Room acoustic effects on monosyllabic word discrimination ability for normal and hearing-impaired children. *Journal of Speech and Hearing Research*, 1978, *21*, 440–448.

under various noise and reverberant conditions. Note that when reverberation and noise are combined, word recognition is reduced markedly. At a S/N ratio of +6 dB, a listening situation commonly found in the classroom setting, word recognition is 60%. When one adds a reverberant condition of only .4 seconds, the mean word recognition is reduced to 52%. At 1.2 seconds, the word recognition score is only 27%. Similar findings have been reported by other investigators (Nabelek & Pickett, 1974a, 1974b; Olsen, 1981).

Acoustic Treatment of Classrooms

The previous discussion has demonstrated that noise levels and prolonged reverberation within the educational environment are usually excessive and can therefore adversely affect a hearing-impaired child's ability to understand speech. Indeed, when new facilities are constructed, special attention should be given to classrooms for hearing-impaired children. Fourcin and coworkers (1980) have discussed in detail the important factors that need consideration in the construction of facilities for the hearing impaired.

The primary difficulty with classrooms, however, is not so much the new facilities, but, rather older classrooms. It is the older vintage schools that usually require the most acoustic treatment for reducing high classroom noise. Room selection is an important factor as a first step in assuring adequate noise levels. To control for external noise, the outside walls should have as few windows as possible, since windows are known to be poor sound insulators. If windows cannot be avoided, a double-paned window with an air space is recommended, in an attempt to produce maximum external noise attenuation. It is also helpful to utilize special landscaping between the classroom and the external noise sources. For example, the use of evergreens or shrubs can help to reduce the noise levels that reach the classroom from the outside (Olsen, 1977).

Numerous examples have been recommended for reducing noise that is generated in the classroom. Some of these noise reduction techniques include: (1) carpeting the classroom and the hallways outside the classroom; (2) using acoustic tile on the ceiling and walls; (3) hanging heavy draperies over the glass windows located on the external walls; (4) lining doors with felt and/or rubber to ensure no acoustic leakage; (5) using felt or rubber caps on chairs and table legs; (6) covering tops of desks with a resilient material such as felt or cork; and (7) recommending rubber-soled shoes for children. Perhaps the most important factor, however, is to select a room that already has excellent acoustics and is not in need of extensive acoustical treatment. For more detail on noise reduction techniques, several sources are recommended (Bess & McConnell, 1981; Finitzo-Hieber, 1982; John & Thomas, 1957; Niemoeller, 1981; Olsen, 1977).

Description of Amplification Systems Used in Education

A summary of the types of amplification systems used most often in education is shown in Table 6-2. These data were taken in a survey of 110 American private and public schools (1,871 classrooms) for the hearing impaired (Sinclair & Freeman, 1981). Note that the majority (91%) of classrooms used personal hearing aids, an FM wireless system, or a combination of the personal hearing aid and an FM wireless device. The remaining 9% of the classrooms were found to utilize personal loops (6%), desk-mounted devices (2%), and induction loop systems (1%). Let us now examine some of these systems used by local educational agencies.

The Personal Hearing Aid

The personal hearing aid is thought to offer a number of advantages particularly when the teacher is working in small group activities where children are functioning independently from the rest of the class. That is, the personal hearing aid is sufficient as long as the distance between the

Table 6-2
Summary of Types of Amplification Systems Currently in Use in American Education

Type of Amplification System	Percentage of Classrooms (N = 1,871)
Personal hearing aid	34
FM-wireless	26
FM-wireless combined with personal hearing aid	31
Personal-loop aid	6
Desk-mounted	2
Room-loop	1

NOTE: From J.S. Sinclair, & B.A. Freeman. The status of classroom amplification in American education. In F.H. Bess, B.A. Freeman, & J.S. Sinclair (Eds.), *Amplification in Education.* Washington, D.C.: The Alexander Graham Bell Association for the Deaf, 1981.

sound source and the pickup microphone does not become too great. These instruments provide excellent mobility, fitting flexibility, child-to-child communication and self-monitoring, signal fidelity, and reasonable stability of performance, provided that the local educational agency offers an ongoing monitoring program. In addition, ear-level hearing aids are now capable of providing the power requirements previously available in only body instruments. The availability of differing types of compression circuitry in personal hearing aids has helped to reduce distortion and has made amplification more acceptable to those individuals with limited dynamic range. Finally, the ear-level hearing aids can provide microphone placement advantages, wearing comfort, and cosmetic appeal for the majority of hearing-impaired children.

Two major problems appear to limit the useful application of a personal hearing aid. First, as noted earlier, the use of this aid as a group system involves a separation between the sound source and the pickup microphone. This distance factor contributes to an unfavorable S/N listening condition, as well as a signal level that may be insufficient to overcome the hearing loss. Generally speaking, however, if the hearing loss does not exceed 90 dB, and the ambient noise level does not exceed 40 dB, a personal hearing aid can be used successfully in the classroom setting (Bess & McConnell, 1981; Boothroyd, 1981). A second problem area with the personal hearing aids is in the reliability and stability of these instruments. Numerous investigators (Bess, 1977; Coleman, 1972; Gaeth & Lounsbury, 1966; Zink, 1972) have noted the high prevalence of malfunctions of personal hearing aids in the schools, especially in those settings where no monitoring program exists.

FM Systems

As a consequence of some of the problems exhibited by personal hearing aids in the classroom setting, educators and audiologists have turned to other educational amplification systems. The FM system reportedly offers some distinct advantages over the personal hearing aid and helps create a better listening condition for the hearing-impaired child. The primary advantage of the FM system is that it affords an acceptable S/N ratio for speech understanding. Traditionally, a transmitter/microphone is worn around the teacher's neck, and a frequency-modulated signal is broadcast to an FM student-receiver unit worn by the child. External receivers coupled to personal earmolds are often used with the student units. The student receivers can additionally provide environmental microphones within the unit, which allow for child-to-child communication, self-monitoring, and general auditory awareness of the classroom environment. The environmental microphones also allow the unit to be used as a personal hearing aid when the FM signal is unavailable. The student receivers can provide internal frequency adjustments and power controls, thus making them more adaptable to a wider range of individual needs. A schematic diagram of a typical FM-transmission system terminating with earphones is shown in Figure 6-3. The FM transmitter converts the audio signal into radio waves that are broadcast into the environment. The signal is picked up by the receiver and converted back into acoustic energy, either at the student's personal hearing aid or at headphones. An example of a typical FM system, including both the transmitter and receivers, is shown in Figure 6-4.

Coupling the Personal Hearing Aid to an FM Unit

A number of newer techniques have been developed for "dovetailing" the personal hearing aid to the FM system (Bess & Gravel, 1981). This concept evolved from an effort to maintain the electroacoustic-response parameters of the personal aid, while at the same time providing the advantages of an improved S/N ratio. The coupling of the hearing aid to

FIGURE 6-3
Simple Schematic Diagram of FM Transmission System Feeding to Headphones

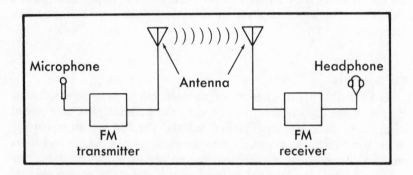

FIGURE 6-4
Example of a Typical FM System, Including Both the Transmitter and Receivers (Courtesy of Phonic Ear)

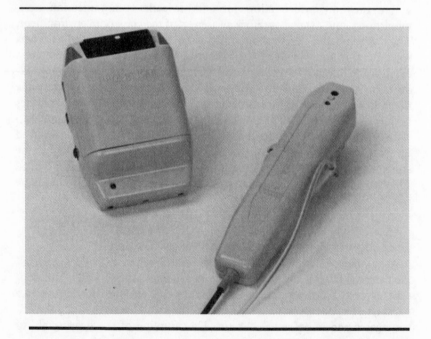

the FM system can be accomplished in three general ways, as shown in Figure 6-5.

1. Electrical Coupling—Electrical coupling (Figure 6-5A) is accomplished by modifying the hearing aid to accept an input jack, or sleeve, that fits over the bottom of the hearing aid. The output voltage of the student-worn FM receiver is then delivered directly to the personal hearing aid. With such an arrangement, three possible input modes are available: (1) for the microphone of the personal hearing aid only; (2) from the input microphone of the FM system only; and (3) a combination of both inputs. The selection of the input modes varies depending upon the specific model and manufacturer. With some hearing aids, the choice of operating modes may be limited to only two conditions (EM, FM, or EM-FM). Furthermore, it should be noted that the modification of the aid may necessitate the elimination of a selection mode. Finally, some of the systems allow the coupling of one or two specific aids only to the FM receiver. While this system does offer unique and flexible options, there are some disadvantages. Some of these disadvantages include system complexity, the need for some instruments to be modified by the manufacturer, and the failure of some of these systems to offer all possible operating modes.

2. Inductive Coupling—The inductive coupling system in Figure 6-5B is comprised of a neck-worn induction loop (mini-loop) that is dovetailed to the student receiver. The FM signal, which is sometimes mixed with an environmental signal within the student receiver, is converted to an electromagnetic field via a wire loop encircling the child's neck. The personal hearing aid is worn in a telecoil position, thereby inductively coupling a hearing aid to the FM receiver/mini-loop combination. Unfortunately, when the hearing aid is switched to the telecoil position, the student's input is limited to auditory signals that are transduced by the teacher's transmitter. Hence, unless the student receiver has environmental microphones, the child is unable to monitor his or her own speech and communicate with peers in the environment. An unknown variable with this type of system is the telecoil response, as well as the consistency and strength of the electromagnetic field encircling the child's head.

3. Acoustic Coupling—Acoustic coupling (Figure 6-5C) is another means of dovetailing the personal hearing aid to the FM receiver. In this system, an acoustic transducer that is electrically coupled to the student receiver is secured to the side of any ear-level case. A piece of flexible tubing from this transducer delivers an acoustic signal to the microphone port of the hearing aid. The microphone opening remains unoccluded and monitoring of environmental sounds is possible when the instrument is set in the microphone position. The transducer can remain on the hearing aid case,

FIGURE 6-5
Illustration of Three Different Approaches for Coupling the Personal Hearing Aid to the FM System (From F. H. Bess and J. S. Gravel. Recent Trends in Educational Amplification. *Hearing Instruments*, **1981,** *32* **(11), 24-29.)**

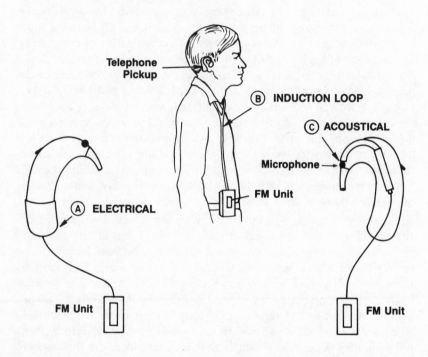

Note: A-electrical coupling; B-inductive coupling; C-acoustical coupling.

while the wire connection to the student FM receiver is detachable. All power limiting, volume control, and frequency response modifications are accomplished by the personal hearing aid and earmold coupling arrangement. If desired, the transducer can be easily removed from one hearing aid and secured to another instrument. It is important to emphasize here that this particular coupling device provides only a mixed FM-environmental microphone signal, and that it is not possible (at this writing) to obtain an FM-only condition. The selection switches on the instrument remain unmodified.

There are some optimal characteristics that seem desirable in these different personal FM systems. First, for the inductive-coupling systems, it would be ideal to know the telecoil sensitivity, as well as some general orientation information. Second, it would be advantageous for any coupling device to provide all three positions on the ear-level instruments. Third, it would be advantageous for these systems to have audio-input capabilities.

Although these coupling systems afford increased flexibility, and, theoretically, the combined advantages of a personal hearing aid and FM system, there is limited information available with regard to the response characteristics, as well as the behavioral performance, of children using these systems. Indeed, the multitude of fitting options and the advantages and disadvantages of these different fittings are areas that are in need of further investigation. Both the teacher and the audiologist must be familiar with the various options available if they hope to capitalize on the benefits that these systems offer.

Infrared System

Infrared systems offer the transmission of signals by means of infrared light. While these systems are not yet used commonly in the schools, they have become popular in many public facilities (e.g., auditoriums) throughout the country. Infrared amplification may also soon gain popularity in the educational setting. With this particular device the teacher utilizes an FM microphone-transmitter, and an FM receiver is attached to the infrared transmitter. The teacher's speech is converted from an acoustic signal to an electrical signal and then modulated into a radio frequency carrier wave by the FM microphone-transmitter. This signal is received by an infrared transmitter that modulates it in infrared light frequencies emitted from radiators. Several light-emitting radiators are usually placed throughout the classroom for uniform distribution. The modulated infrared light is then picked up by a receiver and demodulated before it enters the hearing aid. One modification of this arrangement is to place a dual-channel microphone in the center of the room. The microphone is hard-wired to the infrared transmitter, eliminating the need for the initial FM transmission from the teacher.

Accessory Devices

The personal hearing aid and classroom system do not always provide an adequate solution to a hearing-impaired child's individual amplification needs. Hearing-impaired children, like their normal hearing peers, are exposed to information from a wide variety of sources. The audiologist needs to give consideration to all listening situations encountered by the hearing-impaired child whether it occurs in the classroom or outside the school setting. That is, in meeting the amplification requirements of a hearing-impaired child, the audiologist should be familiar with the available accessory devices. A summary of some of the various supplemental amplification devices that can be useful to hearing-impaired children is shown in Table 6-3.

Personal communication via telephone is an essential means for young people to interact and interexperience. This important means of communication is occasionally overlooked when recommending a personal amplification system. In a recent unpublished survey by the Hearing Industries Association, 55% of the hearing aids sold in 1981 were not equipped with a telecoil. It was also found that hearing aid dispensers seldom counsel families of hearing-impaired children with regard to the desirable type of phone to use in the home. Counseling about phone type seems important, since several styles are not compatible with the telephone induction coil. In addition, a large percentage of personal hearing aids used on children with a mild-to-moderate hearing loss do not have induction coils. For these children, amplifiers are available that can be housed in the telephone receivers with volume controls as well as portable attachments. Recently, an external attachment has been produced that works in conjunction with the hearing aid induction coil. This system provides additional gain and is especially helpful to those students with severe hearing losses. Most of these telephone options are relatively inexpensive and can be most helpful to the hearing impaired.

The increased usage of multi-media in today's educational programming necessitates the consideration of auxiliary options in the selection of an educational system. Some FM teacher transmitter units can receive an auxiliary input from a television set, movie projector, or tape recorder. These options allow for a fidelity input that cannot always be achieved by simply acoustically coupling the microphone to the sound source. Other devices are available that are less expensive than the complete educational amplification system (teacher transmitter/student receiver); however, many of these require a direct connection from the source to the individual.

Even pleasurable events such as vacation trips can be isolating experiences if the hearing-impaired child cannot participate in the interpersonal interactions that occur. Road and wind noises inside an automobile often adversely affect the S/N ratio. Under such conditions, a relatively inexpensive microphone can be dovetailed to the child's personal hearing aid, thus enhancing the S/N ratio. This option should also be considered for teenagers enrolled in driver education. It is simply impossible to speechread and observe the road simultaneously; under such conditions, a fidelity signal is of utmost importance.

It is emphasized here that the child's auditory needs are not simply limited to those hours spent in classroom activities. Within a typical listening day, the hearing-impaired child will be exposed to sundry auditory experiences, many of which will not occur within the classroom but will still play an important role in learning. As audiologists, our goal should be to meet all of these amplification needs of the hearing-impaired, not just some of them (Bliss, Gravel, & Princenthal, 1980; Ross, 1982).

Selection and Evaluation of Educational Systems

Criteria Used in System Selection

When a teacher or audiologist decides to purchase a new educational amplification system, it is important that they develop criteria for selecting the type of hearing aid they desire. Bess and McConnell (1981) have outlined several desirable characteristics for amplification systems used in the educational setting. Some of these include hearing loss suitability, educational suitability, simplicity and reliability, flexibility, and cost effectiveness. Hearing loss suitability simply implies that the hearing aid should be appropriate to the child's hearing loss. Most of the modern systems today allow for this capability; however, there are some FM wireless systems that are limited in terms of altering the response characteristics. Educational suitability means that the amplification unit should at a minimum provide a quality signal in a variety of different educational settings. A desirable educational system would afford a sufficiently loud signal delivered at an acceptable S/N ratio, self-monitoring, child-to-child communication, and the possibility for binaural reception. Simplicity and reliability are features that are often overlooked but are essential if the system is to be used effectively. The units should be simple for teachers of the hearing-impaired to operate, easy to check, and, most importantly, should not require a great deal of maintenance. Perhaps one of the most important criteria in the selection of an instrument is the maintenance required for a given system. Our experience has suggested that maintenance will vary not only as a function of the manufacturer, but also within manufacturing companies. That is, the quality of maintenance will vary in different regions of the country. A reliable system is one that will yield electroacoustic specifications similar to the data reported by the manufacturer. Unfortunately, standardized procedures have not been developed for specifying electroacoustic characteristic procedures. Nevertheless, the consumer should have knowledge of the electroacoustic characteristics the instrument is capable of offering, as well as the measurement procedures employed. Flexibility is certainly a most essential feature in selecting any

Table 6-3
Summary of Accessory Amplification Devices

Input	Device	Description	Advantages	Disadvantages
Telephone	Internal telephone amplifier	Volume control installed by phone company in telephone receiver	Volume control easily adjusted; good range in gain; clear signal	Telephone usage restricted to modified phone; monthly fee; not available on all styles of phones
	External telephone amplifier	Hearing aid telecoil	A personal hearing aid can be used if aid equipped with circuit; adjustable volume control (can also be used with induction-loop systems)	Strength not always dependable; doesn't work on all phone styles
		Small device attaches to phone earpiece (used without hearing aid induction coil)	Portable; adjustable volume control; inexpensive; one-time expense	Battery operated; alignment problems
		Amplifier snaps on to earpiece (operates in conjunction with hearing aid induction coil)	Portable; adjustable gain control; provides extra power when used with hearing aid telecoil; versatile (some models can also be used as a television and radio amplifier)	Battery operated; alignment problems; relatively expensive

Television	Amplifier without a direct connection to source	Loudspeaker	Option for persons who have trouble manipulating T-switch or holding the receiver to aid for any length of time; (provides extra gain without feedback problems when used in addition to one's personal hearing aid)	Limits phone usage to the modified phone
Radio	Same options as television	Induction loop TV/radio kit: Kit includes materials for setting up an induction loop system in home or office (components can also be purchased separately from local TV/radio stores)	Mobility around room; improved signal/noise ratio	Trouble and expense of setting up; must have aid with T-switch; unable to hear environmental sounds
Tape Recorder	Same options as TV and radio	Radio with TV band	Good quality; can be used as radio	Fairly expensive
Signaling Devices	Telephone signal amplifier	Suction cup attaches to surface of phone or doorbell, produces a loud tone	Allows individual to hear phone signal at some distance	Battery operated
Signaling Devices	High intensity doorbell	Large doorbell which provides much greater intensity than standard bells or chimes	Alerts person from some distance away	Installation

system for the educational setting. Flexibility here implies that there be external controls for manipulating electroacoustic characteristics, and that there are several input and output systems available. Recall that flexibility can be affected when an FM system is coupled to some ear-level hearing aids. Finally, this system should be cost effective. That is, the initial cost should be affordable, and the expenses for maintenance and repair should be reasonable. An excellent summary of the general amplification expenses experienced in a large public school audiology program has been reported by Hoversten (1981).

Once we have selected and purchased this system, it is essential to evaluate periodically both the electroacoustic and the behavioral performance of these units. Both the audiologist and educator of the hearing impaired must know that the systems are performing as well or even better than the personal hearing aid alone. Finally, it is important to note that the performance of a system in one mode cannot necessarily be inferred when the system is switched to another mode.

Electroacoustic Assessment

It is essential for the audiologist to analyze electroacoustically both the personal hearing aid and the FM system. At present, however, there exists no satisfactory standard for measuring the electroacoustic characteristics of FM systems. The closest approximation to a workable standard has been the document proposed by the International Electrotechnical Commission (1979). Unfortunately, this proposal fails to identify exact measurement procedures for classroom systems. This does not mean, however, that it is not possible to obtain information with regard to the electroacoustic characteristics of FM systems. Sinclair, Freeman, and Riggs (1981) have recommended an approach similar to the American National Standards Institute (ANSI, 1976) procedures for measuring the electroacoustic performance of personal hearing aids. These procedures can be used on an interim basis, until a standard specific to educational systems is available. Currently, there is an ANSI working group (ANSI SG S3-69) that is charged with developing a standard for measuring the performance of classroom systems.

Behavioral Assessment

Evaluation of the personal hearing aid for a young hearing-impaired child is an intensive and ongoing process. Once a hearing impairment is identified, the audiologist spends a great deal of time selecting an amplification system that best meets the child's needs. Typically, consideration is given to the type of hearing aid arrangement, choice of ear, and the desired electroacoustic characteristics. The performance with the selected hearing aid is then evaluated on a periodic basis, and occasionally the instrument is modified, as more information becomes available about the child's auditory and educational needs. Unfortunately, monitoring and periodic re-evaluation of educational amplification systems does not usually occur (Bess & McConnell, 1981). If it is important for the personal hearing aid, it should be no less important for that system used to assist the child with learning in the classroom. There appear to be two basic factors that have precluded the evaluation of educational amplification systems: (1) educators of the hearing-impaired and educational audiologists are not as knowledgeable about the use and care of these instruments; and (2) no accepted procedure exists for evaluating the behavioral performance of these systems. Whatever the amplification system used by the child, its performance should be evaluated periodically by the audiologist to insure that the instrument(s) is affording adequate auditory input. Although no guidelines are presently available for evaluating FM systems, there are some practical procedures that can be used.

Perhaps the simplest technique is to evaluate the system under actual classroom conditions. For example, a simple speech-recognition test for children (Bess, 1982) can be administered from a specified distance in the classroom. Under such conditions, an FM system can be assessed by comparing the recognition scores obtained under different electroacoustic settings. The EM mode of the FM system and the personal aid can also be evaluated in this manner. When one compares the performance of an FM trainer to the personal hearing aid, the differences in speech-recognition improvement are usually quite marked. That is, the FM system ordinarily will provide much better speech understanding (10 - 60%) than the personal hearing aid (Ross, Brackett, & Maxon, 1982).

It is also feasible with some systems to obtain a soundfield audiogram with and without the FM trainer. A test arrangement that can be used to obtain a soundfield audiogram with an FM system is shown in Figure 6-6. In this example, the FM transmitter is located on a stand 30 cm from the speaker. Prior to testing, the field is specified at a distance of 30 cm for narrow bands of noise (250-6 kHz). Towards this end, sound pressure levels (SPL) are measured for each test frequency at various hearing level-attenuator settings. The child is then seated 2 meters from the speaker. After obtaining unaided thresholds, functional gain measurements can be obtained for the personal hearing aid, the FM system in the EM mode, and FM system in the FM mode. An illustration of actual data measured under these conditions is shown in Figure 6-7. The bottom curve (triangles) depicts normal hearing threshold sensitivity, whereas the top curve (squares)

FIGURE 6-6
Test Arrangement for Obtaining a Soundfield Audiogram with an FM System

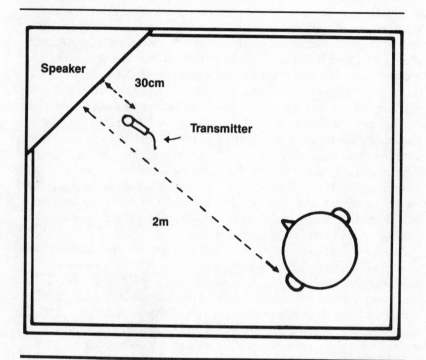

represents the unaided threshold measurements of the hearing-impaired subject. The shaded area comprises the approximate boundaries for the spectrum of conversational speech. The three curves in the center show the aided responses for the personal hearing aid (A), the FM trainer in the EM mode (E), and the FM trainer in the FM mode (F). The differences between curves (A) (E) and curve (F) reflect, in part, differences in distance between the sound source and the microphone. Note that the performance for the personal hearing aid and the FM trainer in the EM mode is similar across all test frequencies. With this measurement procedure, it is possible to compare the soundfield performance among several FM systems, looking at both the EM and FM modes. The reader is cautioned at this point that FM trainers, as they presently exist, were not designed specifically for this type of soundfield measurement. That is, some manufacturers have designed their transmitters such that there is a lower limit-input level. Hence, when the intensity of the input is less than this lower limit, the transmitter

FIGURE 6-7
Illustration of Sound Field Data That Can be Obtained in the Assessment of an FM System

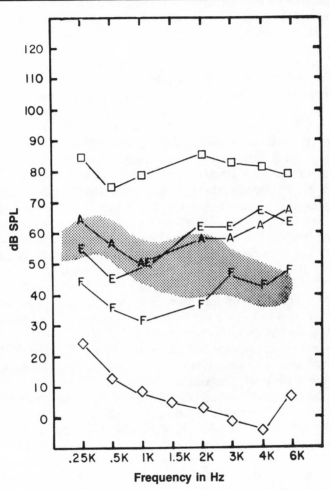

Note: The bottom curve (triangles) depicts normal hearing, and the top curve (squares) represents unaided thresholds for a hearing-impaired subject. The shaded area comprises the boundaries for the spectrum of conversational speech. The curves in the center show aided responses for the personal aid (A), the FM trainer in the EM mode (E), and the FM trainer in the FM mode (F).

output is automatically shut off. Since the lower limit level may vary from one manufacturer to the next, it is simply not possible to obtain sound-field audiograms on some transmitters, whereas, with other systems, there will be limitations due to the degree of hearing impairment. Consequently, the soundfield technique is most valuable for children with severe-to-profound hearing losses.

Monitoring Amplification in Education

Reference has been made on several occasions in this chapter to the fact that hearing aids worn by children in the schools do not always work properly. Such a finding implies that it is important for us to develop monitoring systems that will help to eliminate the problem of poorly functioning hearing aids. At a minimum, maintenance programs should consist of education of parents and teachers on the use and care of the hearing aid, a daily visual and listening examination, monthly electroacoustic checks, and comprehensive physical inspections (Bess & McConnell, 1981). Perhaps the most important feature of any amplification-monitoring program is educating the parent and teacher to trouble-shoot an amplification system. Toward this end, each parent and teacher should be provided with a trouble-shooting kit that can be used to conduct daily inspections of the hearing aid. The traditional trouble-shooting kit includes the following basic ingredients: (1) a drying agent for removing moisture; (2) pipe cleaners; (3) a battery tester; (4) a hearing aid stethoscope; (5) pencil-style typewriter eraser; (6) spare batteries; (7) extra cords; and (8) an extra receiver. The visual component of the inspection process involves checking controls to ensure proper external settings, checking and cleaning the microphone aperture with the bristle brush, checking the receiver for cracks or other defects, checking the earmold for rough edges, cracks, or cerumen, checking the battery contacts for corrosion and dirt, and testing the battery voltage. A listening check should also be conducted using the hearing aid stethoscope. With the amplification system set at an "as worn" condition, the audiologist can subjectively check the hearing aid for distortion, feedback problems, and adequacy of the volume control. For a comprehensive review of monitoring techniques and procedures, the reader is referred elsewhere (Bess & McConnell, 1981; Hanners & Sitton, 1974; Hoversten, 1981; Musket, 1982; Ross, Brackett, & Maxon, 1982).

Status of Amplification in Education

We have already emphasized the importance of amplification in the development of language and learning. It is almost superfluous to note at this point that a classroom teacher's efforts will be to no avail if the student is unable to hear or understand because of an inadequate signal. Indeed, amplification systems used in the educational setting are important tools in the provision of a quality education for the hearing-impaired child. Let us now examine the status of systems available to the hearing-impaired child under actual classroom conditions. Prior to looking at the performance characteristics of hearing aids in the schools, it is appropriate to examine the extent to which these systems are used in education.

Use of Amplification in the Schools

In a survey of 997 hearing-impaired students, Karchmer and Kirwin (1977) reported that almost 80% were found to use a personal hearing aid or group-type system in the classroom at least part of the time. Karchmer and Kirwin also reported that hearing aid use varies as a function of hearing level in the better ear. Interestingly, the largest percentage of nonwearers fell into the mild hearing-loss category ($\leq$40 dB) and the profound hearing-loss group ($\geq$91 dB), whereas the highest percentage of hearing aid use was found in students in the moderate-to-severe hearing-loss range (41-90 dB). Other findings of interest included the following: (1) the percentage of hearing aid use decreases with increasing age; and (2) the percentage of hearing aid use increases as family income increases. Shepard, Gorga, Davis, and Stelmachowicz (1981) surveyed the extent of hearing aid use in the Iowa schools and also noted that the lowest percentage of users fell into the mild and profound hearing-loss categories. In addition, these investigators reported that only 1% of their sample (N = 1,250) were using group-type amplification systems. This finding is in sharp contrast to the survey conducted by Sinclair and Freeman (1981), in which 66% of the programs reportedly used group-type systems.

Performance Characteristics

Personal Hearing Aid. For several years now it has been recognized that personal hearing aids worn by hearing-impaired children in the schools do not perform optimally about 50% of the time. Gaeth and Lounsbury (1966) conducted the first comprehensive study on the performance of hearing aids of 134 hearing-impaired children in a regular classroom setting. They reported that at least half of the children were not receiving maximum benefit from their hearing aids. Gaeth and Lounsbury also found that parents had limited knowledge about the use and care of their child's amplification system. Coleman (1972) demonstrated that the instability of hearing aids was also evident in preschool programs for hearing-impaired children. Coleman reported that 50% of the hearing aids were either not functioning or functioning improperly. These two studies, as well as several others (Findlay & Winchester, 1973; Northern, McChord, Fischer, & Evans, 1972; Zink, 1972), clearly demonstrated the need for audiologists, educators, and parents to devote more attention to assuring that hearing-impaired children receive an adequate auditory signal. Consequently, school systems began to obtain the services of educational audiologists for the purpose of evaluating, monitoring, and managing the auditory requirements of hearing-impaired children. Even with the increased usage of audiologists in the school system, however, the performance of hearing aids in the schools remained a problem.

Eleven years following the Gaeth and Lounsbury report, Bess (1977) conducted a study that involved the physical inspection and electroacoustic measurement of randomly selected hearing aids worn by hearing-impaired children in a large metropolitan school system. The educational agency employed a staff of audiologists who reportedly provided comprehensive audiological services to every hearing-impaired child enrolled in the hearing-impaired program. As part of the physical inspection phase, 27% of the 121 hearing aids evaluated were found to have at least one faulty component. Of this 27%, 30% of the ear-level hearing aids had poor tubing, 5% had broken or cracked cases, and 8% of the earmolds were cracked or occluded. Nine percent of the body-worn hearing aids had broken or cracked receivers, and 14% of the cords were judged as inadequate. When batteries were tested for voltage, only 15% were considered weak. Although not considered adequate, these findings represented an improvement from those reported by previous investigators.

• The children's aids were also evaluated electroacoustically for total harmonic distortion (THD) and acoustic gain. The total harmonic distortion measures for the "as worn" and "standard" conditions were computed for 500, 700, and 900 Hz. Seventy-four percent of the hearing aids exhibited an average THD of $\geq 10\%$ for the "standard" measure and 27% of the hearing aids in the "as worn" condition showed total harmonic distortion of $\geq 10\%$. Acoustic gain at 500, 1000, and 2000 Hz was averaged also for the "as worn" and "standard" conditions for the 121 hearing aids. Interestingly, more than 40% of the hearing aids exhibited gain levels of 40 dB or less. According to Bess, many of the children with severe hearing losses were using inappropriate gain levels for the degree of hearing impairment.

It became evident that the management of the child's hearing aid had to go beyond the educational audiologist, specifically those individuals who were important in the child's auditory development. In a field study described by Kemker, McConnell, Logan, and Green (1979), the percentage of malfunctions was reduced by 50%, primarily as a result of enlisting the help of the classroom teacher and/or aide in addition to the audiologist's weekly checks. Hanners and Sitton (1974) introduced a parent-training program designed to familiarize parents with the effects of malfunctioning hearing aids on the auditory signal, knowledge of the hearing aid system, and a systematic approach to monitoring hearing aid performance. Hoversten (1981) took the monitoring process one step further by involving the hearing-impaired students in part of the monitoring process. It is reasoned that if the audiologist is to be an effective advocate of the hearing-impaired child, they must enlist the services of all persons involved with the hearing-impaired child. The audiologist must promote the necessity of appropriate and consistent amplification to the teachers, principals, and parents through in-service training, demonstrations, and programmed materials.

Classroom Amplification Systems. It has long been assumed that FM systems provide several advantages over the personal hearing aid. Some of the stated advantages include better stability, reliability, and an overall improvement in the quality of the speech signal. Unfortunately, the limited data available on this topic does not support such an assumption. In fact, the status of classroom amplification systems does not appear to be any better than what has been found with personal hearing aids.

Hoversten (1981) reported that of 532 classroom amplification units in use for the 1978-79 school year, 149 (28%) required repair during the school year. A mean of 24 days was required for repair. Hoversten also reported that the average cost of repair per unit was over $28, however, the average annual maintenance cost was $13.36 per piece of equipment used. According to the audiologists in the system, the most frequent problems were dead batteries and poor battery contacts. Intermittency and feedback problems were the most common concerns of the teachers.

In another study, Sinclair, Bess, and Riggs (1981) examined the physical and electroacoustic characteristics of 89 student receiver units and 28 teacher microphone/transmitter units used in a large metropolitan school system. At least half of the student and teacher units were found negligent in one category of physical inspection. For the student units, the greatest percentage of problems was found in the receivers and cords. Broken antennae were the major defects in the teacher units. Even with the number of physical problems present, however, the units were functional for one ear in at least 97% of the systems.

Several investigators have evaluated the performance characteristics of classroom amplification systems under laboratory conditions. In the field study reported above, measurements of saturation output, gain, total harmonic distortion, and internal noise output were performed on all units in the "as worn" and "full on" volume settings. The median high-frequency average saturation output was 134 dB SPL, and the gain measurements ranged from 30 to 70 dB. Further, total harmonic distortion was found to be very low. Sinclair et al. (1981) also analyzed the amount of gain provided by the FM systems as a function of the child's hearing loss. Interestingly, there appeared to be no relationship between the amount of full-on or as-worn gain to the degree of hearing loss.

Freeman, Sinclair, and Riggs (1980) evaluated eight FM units from four different manufacturers. In general, differences were found in gain between the EM and FM modes at different settings on the volume control dial. It was evident that the output of one mode could not be used to predict performance in the other.

Freeman and coworkers also examined the internal noise levels produced by the FM wireless units in EM and FM modes. More than half of the units exhibited over 90 dB SPL of continuous noise when the unit was full on. All the receivers produced greater levels of noise output in the FM mode, as compared to EM.

It was noted earlier that the performance characteristics of dovetailing techniques are essentially unexplored. A recent study by Gravel (1982) highlighted some of the potential problems with the inductive coupling systems. Gravel found that the response varies as a function of head orientation. An example of this variation in hearing aid response is shown in Figure 6-8.

This figure represents the averaged output-response characteristics obtained on KEMAR for a hearing aid inductively coupled to a personal FM system. In this example, the selection switch on an earlevel hearing aid located on KEMAR's left ear, was set to the "T" (telecoil) position. The teleloop was placed around KEMAR's neck, and the attached FM receiver unit was located at the manikin's torso. The volume control of the hearing aid was adjusted to achieve the reference test gain position (RTG) re: the previously obtained SSPL 90 measuremment. For both the RTG and Full on Gain measurements, a 60 dB input was held constant at the FM transmitter microphone via a miniature control microphone located ±4 mm from the port opening. The transmitter unit assembly was positioned one meter away from the receiver unit on KEMAR. Signals were introduced into the soundfield via a speaker.

The solid line represents averaged output for 10 discrete frequencies averaged over two runs, with KEMAR's head at 0° (directly forward). The

FIGURE 6-8
Averaged Output Response Characteristics Obtained on KEMAR
for a Hearing Aid Inductively Coupled to a Personal FM System

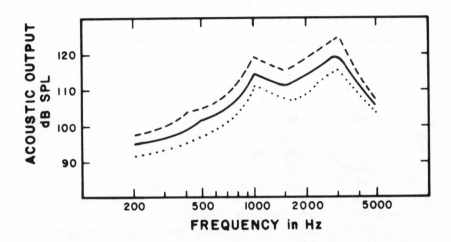

Note: Solid line represents output with KEMAR's head at 0°
(directly in front of sound field speaker), whereas the dotted and
dashed lines show the output obtained when the head is oriented
at ±45°.

dotted line represents the output measured with KEMAR's head oriented
at +45°, while the hearing aid volume control remained unchanged.
Similarly, the dashed line denotes the averaged output at -45° head position. Differences in output for this example were as great as 9 dB across
the three head positions. Such head orientation variations (telecoil position variations) within the teleloop were evident in varying degrees for both
RTG and Full on Gain measurements across all hearing aids (3) and FM
teleloop systems (2) evaluated. Substantial variations in SSPL 90
measurements were also obtained for some hearing aid-teleloop combinations. Indeed, there is an essential need to obtain additional information
on the performance characteristics of other coupling systems.

It should be evident from this review that the use of an FM unit does
not automatically guarantee a problem-free system. The data on performance characteristics highlights the need for audiologists and teachers to

monitor these systems on a periodic basis, just as we do with personal hearing aids.

Afterword

In this chapter we have reviewed and discussed some of the important aspects of amplification in the educational setting. It should seem obvious from this review that there is considerable room for us to improve our current efforts of affording amplification to hearing-impaired children in the schools. The importance of the classroom environment to the hearing-impaired child was emphasized. It is strongly believed that present-day group-type systems offer definite advantages over the personal hearing aid, and that these systems can be of considerable educational value to many hearing-impaired children. Audiologists and educators, however, must improve their efforts to monitor and maintain educational amplification if we expect to realize fully the benefit of this form of amplification. There is also a need for a greater awareness of the importance and value of educational systems by all individuals who come in contact with hearing-impaired children. Finally, there is an urgent need to increase the research activity associated with educational amplification, as well as develop new and innovative electroacoustic and behavioral assessment procedures. We simply cannot afford to do less.

Acknowledgments

The authors wish to express their gratitude to Barb Coulson for typing the manuscript and to Don Riggs for preparing the figures. We are also grateful to Judy Gravel for her assistance in the preparation of this manuscript.

References

American National Standards Institute. Specification of hearing aid characteristics (S3.22-1976). New York: American National Standards Institute, 1976.

Bess, F.H. Condition of hearing aids worn by children in a public school setting. In *The condition of hearing aids worn by children in a public school program.* HEW Publication No. (OE) 77-05002, 1977, 13-23.

Bess, F.H. Clincial assessment of speech recognition. In D.F. Konkle & W.F. Rintelmann (Eds.), *Principles of speech audiometry.* Baltimore: University Park Press, 1982.

Bess, F.H., & McConnell, F.E. *Audiology, education and the hearing impaired child.* St. Louis: C.V. Mosby, 1981.

Bess, F.H., & Gravel, J.S. Recent trends in educational amplification. *Hearing Instruments,* 1981, *32,* (11), 24-29.

Bliss, T., Gravel, J., & Princenthal, D. Mainstreaming in the theater. *Hearing Instruments,* 1980, *31,* (4), 15-16.

Boothroyd, A. Group hearing aids. In F.H. Bess, B.A. Freeman, & J.S. Sinclair (Eds.), *Amplification in education.* Washington, DC: The Alexander Graham Bell Association for the Deaf, 1981.

Coleman, R.F. Stability of children's hearing aids in an acoustic preschool. Final report, HEW, U.S. Office of Education, National Center for Educational Research and Development, 522466, 1972.

Findlay, R.C., & Winchester, R.A. Defects in hearing aids worn by preschool and school age children. Paper presented at the American Speech-Language-Hearing Association Convention, Detroit, November, 1973.

Finitzo-Hieber, T. Classroom acoustics. In R.J. Roeser, & M.P. Downs, (Eds.), *Auditory disorders in school children.* New York: Thieme-Stratton, 1982.

Finitzo-Hieber, T., & Tillman, T.W. Room acoustic effects on monosyllabic word discrimination ability for normal and hearing impaired children. *Journal of Speech and Hearing Research,* 1978, *21,* 440-448.

Fourcin, A.J., Joy, D., Kennedy, M. et al. Design for educational facilities for deaf children. *British Journal of Audiology,* Supplement No. 3, 1980.

Freeman, B.A., Sinclair, J.S., & Riggs, D.E. Electroacoustic performance characteristics of FM auditory trainers. *Journal of Speech and Hearing Disorders,* 1980, *45,* 16-26.

Gaeth, J.H., & Lounsbury, E. Hearing aids and children in elementary schools. *Journal of Speech and Hearing Disorders,* 1966, *31,* 289-293.

Gengel, R.W. Acceptable speech-to-noise ratios for aided speech discrimination by the hearing impaired. *Journal of Auditory Research,* 1971, *11,* 219-222.

Glorig, A. *Noise and your ear.* New York: Grune & Stratton, 1958.

Gravel, J. Unpublished study, Vanderbilt University, 1982.

Hanners, B.A., & Sitton, A.B. Ears to hear: A daily hearing aid monitoring program. *The Volta Review,* 1974, *76,* 530-536.

Hoversten, G. A public school audiology program: Amplification maintenance, auditory management, and inservice education. In F.H. Bess, B.A. Freeman, & J.S. Sinclair (Eds.), *Amplification in education.* Washington, DC: The Alexander Graham Bell Association for the Deaf, 1981.

International Electrotechnical Commission. Methods of measurement of electroacoustical characteristics of hearing aids. Part III. Hearing aid equipment not entirely worn on the listener (IEC Pub. 118-3-1979). Geneva, Switzerland: International Electrotechnical Commission, 1979.

John, J.E.J., & Thomas, H. Design and construction of schools for the deaf. In A.W.G. Ewing (Ed.), *Educational guidance and the deaf child.* Washington, DC: *The Volta Review,* 1957.

Karchmer, M.A. & Kirwin, L.A. The use of hearing aids by hearing impaired students in the United States. Office of Demographic Studies Publication, 1977, Series S, Number 2.

Kemker, J.F., McConnell, F., Logan, S.A., & Green, B.W. A field study of children's hearing aids in a school environment. *Language, Speech and Hearing Services in the Schools,* 1979, *10,* 47-53.

Musket, C.H. Maintenance of personal hearing aids. In R.J. Roeser, & M.P. Downs, (Eds.), *Auditory disorders in school children.* New York: Thieme-Stratton, 1982.

Nabalek, A.K., & Pickett, J.M. Monaural and binaural speech perception through hearing aids under noise and reverberation with normal and hearing impaired listeners. *Journal of Speech and Hearing Research,* 1974, *17,* 724-739. (a)

Nabalek, A.K., & Pickett, J.M. Reception of consonants in a classroom as affected by monaural and binaural listening, noise, reverberation and hearing aids. *Journal of the Acoustical Society of America,* 1974, *56,* 628-639. (b)

Niemoller, A. Physical concepts of speech communication in classrooms for the deaf. In F.H. Bess, B.A. Freeman, & J.S. Sinclair (Eds.), *Amplification in education.* Washington, DC: The Alexander Graham Bell Association for the Deaf, 1981.

Northern, J.L., McChord, W., Fischer, E., & Evans, P. Hearing services in residential schools for the deaf. *Maico Audiology Library Series,* 1978, *1* (2).

Olsen, W.O. Acoustics and amplification in classrooms for the hearing impaired. In F.H. Bess (Ed.), *Childhood deafness: Causation, assessment and management.* New York: Grune & Stratton, 1977.

Olsen, W.O. The effects of noise and reverberation on speech intelligibility. In F.H. Bess, B.A. Freeman, & J.S. Sinclair (Eds.), *Amplification in education.* Washington, DC: The Alexander Graham Bell Association for the Deaf, 1981.

Pearsons, K.S., Bennett, R.L., & Fidell, S. Speech levels in various noise environments. Office of Health and Ecological Effects. U.S. Environmental Protection Agency, EFA-600/1-77-025, Washington, DC, May, 1977.

Ross, M. Communication access. In G. Studebaker & F.H. Bess (Eds.). The Vanderbilt Hearing Aid Report. *Monographs in Contemporary Audiology.* Upper Darby, PA: Educational Services Division, Instrument Associates Inc., 1982.

Ross, M., Brackett, D., & Maxon, A. *Hard of hearing children in regular schools.* Englewood Cliffs, NJ: Prentice-Hall, 1982.

Sabine, H.J. Acoustical materials. In C.M. Harris (Ed.), *Handbook of noise control.* New York: McGraw-Hill, 1957.

Sanders, D. Noise conditions in normal school classrooms. *Journal of Exceptional Children,* 1965, *31,* 344-353.

Shepard, N.T., Gorga, M.P., Davis, J.M., & Stelmachowicz, P.G. Characteristics of hearing-impaired children in the public schools: Part I—Demographic data. *Journal of Speech and Hearing Disorders,* 1981, *46,* 123-129.

Sinclair, S., Bess, F.H., & Riggs, D.E. A field study of FM-wireless amplification in hearing-impaired classrooms. Paper presented at the American Speech-Language-Hearing Association Convention, Los Angeles, November, 1981.

Sinclair, S., & Freeman, B.A. The status of classroom amplification in American education. In F.H. Bess, B.A. Freeman, & J.S. Sinclair (Eds.), *Amplification in education.* Washington, DC: The Alexander Graham Bell Association for the Deaf, 1981.

Sinclair, S., Freeman, B.A., & Riggs, D.E. The use of the hearing aid test box to assess the performance of FM auditory training units. In F.H. Bess, B.A. Freeman, & J.S. Sinclair (Eds.), *Amplification in education.* Washington, DC: The Alexander Graham Bell Association for the Deaf, 1981.

Zink, G.D., Hearing aids children wear: A longitudinal study of performance. *The Volta Review,* 1972, *74,* 41-51.

Rebecca M. Fischer

Habilitation of the Hearing-Impaired Child

Providing excellent habilitative services for the hearing-impaired child and family continues to present a challenge to audiologists, educators, and speech pathologists. The deficits imposed by impaired hearing are manifested most clearly in the inadequate communication skills of the hearing impaired, yet have important implications for the development of social, academic, and vocational skills as well. Despite innovations in instructional materials and services, few hearing-impaired students graduate from educational programs with the competencies necessary to confront the complexities of adult life. In a study of the educational achievement of hearing-impaired students, Trybus and Karchmer (1977) reported the reading comprehension and math computation scores of hearing-impaired children aged 8 to 20 as measured by the Special Edition for Hearing Impaired Students of the 1973 Stanford Achievement Test. With respect to reading comprehension, a grade-equivalent score of 4.5 was achieved by half of the students aged 20, while median grade-equivalent scores for math computation were 8.1. The "substantial educational disadvantage" suffered by hearing-impaired graduates as compared to their hearing peers is underlined by these achievement scores, and the inability of half of the 20-year-olds to read at newspaper literacy level emphasizes the failure of the educational system to meet even the minimal language needs of these students.

Numerous assessment tools, language programs, and content area curricula are available to assist the teacher in developing effective strategies for educating the hearing-impaired child. Yet, with few exceptions, research studies confront professionals with a single realization: Despite advances in amplification, improvements in teacher training programs, and rapid developments in language theory, the majority of hearing-impaired children continue to function at a level far below that of their hearing peers.

Few guidelines are available to assist the clinician and family in making decisions regarding instructional programs and diagnostic procedures. Educators are confronted with many curricula for developing language, speech, and reading, and a variety of placement options in which to achieve these competencies. Structured language, programmed language, natural language, and developmental language approaches each appear to have a measure of success with some hearing-impaired children, as do phonetic and phonologic programs for speech development, and wholeword and phonetic methods for teaching reading. Hearing-impaired students may be educated via partial or fulltime integration in regular classrooms in addition to residential facilities and self-contained classrooms. Yet, there is little hard data to help professionals choose the correct combination of programs for each hearing-impaired child. Decisions regarding programming often reflect basic philosophical differences among professionals rather than sensitivity to individual differences in the deaf population. Nowhere is this more evident than in the continuing controversy over communication methodology.

In addition, little information exists on the accuracy of any evaluation tools with respect to the hearing-impaired child, and few instruments have been designed specifically for the hearing impaired, compelling psychologists and educators to interpret the results of tests originally devised for other populations. Thus, the familiarity of the professional with deaf children and their performance on tests is crucial in obtaining accurate estimates of learning potential.

Some recent developments in deaf education have had a positive influence on habilitation procedures, suggesting that a greater number of future graduates from programs may have the necessary academic and communication skills. One of the most far-reaching developments in the field has been the establishment of parent/infant programs, which enabled professionals to offer support and guidance to families of deaf children 0-3. The realization that the early period of life was a crucial language-learning time prompted professionals to devise curricula to take advantage of naturally occurring language-learning opportunities in the home, assisting parents in capitalizing on these events to create a warm communicative environment with the hearing-impaired child.

The expansion of habilitative services offered hearing-impaired children has also been due in part to provisions of Public Law 94-142, the Education for All Handicapped Children Act (1975). Although the law will be discussed in greater detail in the following chapter, a brief review is pertinent to understanding some of the recent developments in education. The federal legislation guaranteed a free appropriate public school education to each handicapped child, and local school systems were held responsible for delivering services to certified students. PL 94-142 required that an individualized education program (IEP) addressing instructional needs be developed for every handicapped child. To be included in the program were (1) the child's current level of performance, (2) a statement of annual goals, and (3) objective criteria for evaluating the child's performance and achievement of the designated objectives (Dublinske, 1978). A second important provision mandated that, when appropriate, handicapped children receive their education with normally functioning students. This concept of "least restrictive environment" encouraged educators to integrate students and to provide options for placement, including self-contained, resource, and mainstreamed classrooms.

Coincidentally with the passage of this act, a larger proportion of hearing-impaired children were being instructed in local educational settings than at any previous time. A national survey conducted in 1974-1975 by Rawlings and Trybus (1978) indicated that approximately two-thirds of all hearing-impaired students attended day schools and special classes, as opposed to residential facilities. Thus, a greater number of professionals in local communities were providing services for hearing-impaired children and were accountable for designing and evaluating individual instructional plans.

This chapter will examine some of the current practices employed in the habilitation of hearing-impaired children. The development of communication skills will be explored and methodological issues discussed. Assessment procedures and placement options will be described, and guidelines for programming habilitative services suggested.

The Development of Communication Skills

In examining communication development in the normally hearing infant and preschooler, one cannot help but marvel at the apparent ease with which skills are acquired and the linguistic proficiency of very young hearing children. Experience with special populations only increases appreciation for the enormity of the language-learning task. The knowledge that language is learned rather than taught may provide guidance for improving current procedures for developing language facility and communication competence in the hearing impaired.

Hearing impairment exerts a profound effect on all aspects of language learning including syntax, semantics, and pragmatics. However, until recently researchers have focused on describing the syntax and vocabulary of hearing-impaired children. The hearing-impaired child appears to be deficient in the use of all word classes, but especially structural components or function words. Studies of vocabulary and lexical items reveal that the deaf possess a basic vocabulary, but fail to expand and develop the nuances and variations in meaning. In addition, words are often locked into a rigid syntactic frame characterized by short simple active declarative sentences. Studies by Quigley and associates (Quigley, Power, & Steinkamp, 1977) described in depth the emergence of syntactic rules in the language of the hearing impaired. Results indicated that the hierarchy of difficulty with respect to syntactic structures was similar though not identical for deaf and hearing students. However, while hearing children had mastered the majority of syntactic rules by age 8, only syntactic rules pertaining to negation, conjunctions, and questions had been well established for even the oldest hearing-impaired students.

Language Habilitation

Traditionally, language-teaching methods have emphasized syntactic development and focused on surface structure forms. For example, the Fitzgerald Key (Fitzgerald, 1949), which is still used by many classroom teachers to develop language, served as a visual representation of spoken English. Six columns designating parts of speech assisted the child in formulating sentences by serving as a reference for sentence construction. Although Fitzgerald emphasized that the Key was designed to reinforce language patterns produced in the classroom, too few teachers and clinicians provided those experiences for the hearing-impaired language learner. Instead, the Key became the primary source of language input. The use of structured language approaches such as the Key and Apple Tree (1975), without establishing a semantic and pragmatic basis for language, produces some of the syntactic errors typical of deaf language and is partly responsible for some of the communication deficiencies described earlier. The natural approach (Groht, 1958) emphasized the development of language within meaningful communication situations and stressed semantic and communication competence. Groht believed that language was best learned when the child required language to express immediate wants or needs. Normal language development principles were stressed by Groht, but oftentimes, in practice, teachers with limited information failed to utilize a developmental approach, and teaching became haphazard and ineffective.

Perhaps most frustrating and detrimental to providing a quality language program for hearing-impaired children is the failure of many programs to establish a curriculum or philosophy of language development. Programs utilizing a structured or natural approach are uncertain as to the order of language development. In addition, many of the tools best designed to provide additional support for the understanding of written language are instead used as the basis for developing oral/signed English, without the teacher first establishing a reason for using those particular structures. In other words, the reinforcement rather than the language experience itself serves as the basis for language acquisition. This certainly is in contrast to what we know about language development in normal-hearing children, and it presumes that the hearing impaired are programmed quite differently for language learning, that is, that they learn language almost as an academic exercise, rather than as a tool for communication.

Fortunately, we are now beginning to recognize that for both language and speech to be effectively utilized, each must occur in the context of the child's environment, and must develop as the result of an idea or desire the child wishes to express. In other words, meaning or semantics, rather than syntax, dominates language acquisition. Syntactic theories have given way to linguistic theories. One such curriculum of instruction has been designed by Blackwell, Engen, Fischgrund, and Zarcadoolas (1978), which emphasizes a linguistic approach and focuses on five basic sentence patterns from which other linguistic patterns are developed.

Others have turned instead to theories of conversational development—how the child learns to communicate within the context of a dialogue. From normal-hearing children we know that preverbal children develop the idea of turn taking or shared conversation through daily interaction with close family members. Later, the child learns to use language to express wants, gain information, question, etc. We see that the need to communicate motivates semantic development, which, in turn, also provides the impetus for the development of complex syntactic structures as communication desires become more complex. In contrast, much of our teaching with hearing-impaired children begins with vocabulary lists and imposes language upon the child from an adult viewpoint.

Kretschmer (1982) suggests that we look at "discourse teaching" rather than "sentence production teaching," and focus first on the overall format or function of a communication situation and then on how the child selects the right words and sentence structures so that the sentences relate to each other and form a cohesive group. Rarely, except in spelling exercises or grammatical practice, does the normal-hearing child write individual sentences. Unfortunately it is just the opposite with the hearing-impaired child. Kretschmer also suggests teaching grammar meaningfully through conversations or story formats—that there is a relationship between format and grammar.

We are beginning to realize that language grows out of communication situations, and that the need to communicate must be stressed, rather than syntactic structure. Although this area of research and curriculum design is just opening up, it promises to offer teachers new and exciting methods of helping the hearing-impaired child to learn language.

Speech Development

One cannot deny that we live in a world which communicates a vast amount of information orally, in personal conversations, small group interactions, classroom dialogues, and in the dissemination of ideas through mass media such as television and radio. Because of this dependence on verbal communication, intelligible speech is important for all hearing-impaired children, regardless of the communication method employed. The ability to receive and produce speech offers the hearing-impaired child wide exposure to ideas and the opportunity to exchange opinions.

Thus, it is somewhat ironic that the ability of the average hearing-impaired child to communicate orally has changed very little over the past 50 years. Contemporary research reiterates the findings of previous studies, which showed that the speech of hearing-impaired individuals was characterized by faulty production of both prosodic and articulatory features, specifically poor rhythmical patterns such as slow rate of production, frequent pauses, and poor differentiation of stressed and unstressed syllables; atypical voice quality including faulty pitch and intonation, nasality, and breathiness; prolongation, neutralization, and diphthongization of vowels; and substitution, omission, and poor articulation of consonants. Despite increased knowledge in speech science and technological advances in rehabilitation and education, our ability to develop effective programs for teaching speech to the hearing impaired has shown little improvement.

Although several methods have been used successfully for a number of years by experienced teachers (Calvert & Silverman, 1975; Clarke School for the Deaf, 1971; Haycock, 1933; Rowe, 1974), a detailed comprehensive design which includes an evaluation procedure, a hierarchy of speech objectives, and specific suggestions for remediation was not available.

Such a program was developed by Ling (1975) and combines the author's own ideas with the features of other speech methods. Perhaps most importantly, Ling developed a sequential system for teaching individual speech phonemes and prosodic features. The program has been widely adopted by individual therapists and teachers utilizing auditory/oral and total communication methods of instruction.

Based upon theoretical evidence in the fields of speech production and acoustic phonetics, the program emphasized speech teaching at the phonetic and phonological levels. A seven-step hierarchy provided a sequential plan for speech habilitation: voicing; suprasegmental features including pitch, duration, and intensity; vowels; consonants by manner, place, and voicing; and blends. At the phonetic level, speech teaching was directed toward developing automaticity through a series of suggested subskills. By emphasizing automatic production through babbled practice with nonsense syllables, the hearing-impaired child was offered an opportunity to rehearse phonemes much as a young baby does. As a result, rate and durational features, as well as individual phonemes, would be produced accurately, thus facilitating generalization into words, phrases, and sentences at the phonological level. Early work was directed toward establishing abundant vocalization and appropriate suprasegmental features, thus avoiding the rehearsal of faulty voice patterns which are difficult to remediate. The program outlined the use of appropriate modalities (audition, vision, and taction) for eliciting speech targets and stressed the utilization of residual hearing as a primary means for recognizing and interpreting speech signals. Ling emphasized that speech teaching should be an efficient, orderly process, allowing the child to progress at a steady pace.

Communication Methodologies

The controversy over communication methodologies continues to divide the professional community working with hearing-impaired children. Individual case histories, descriptive studies, and ex post facto experiments have described the merits of an auditory approach (Ling, Leckie, Pollack, Simser, & Smith, 1981; Milne & Ling, 1981), multi-sensory programs (Geers & Moog, 1978), cued speech (Nicholls, 1979), and total communication (Vernon & Koh, 1970). Although these studies are often cited as evidence of the superiority of one method or philosophy over another, little evidence exists to support such claims. Examination of the research reveals that it is impossible to control the internal and external variables which affect a child's educational performance, for example, family support, intellectual capacity, the integrity of the central nervous system, socio-economic factors, hearing loss, and, perhaps most importantly, program quality. The result of the debate has been to distract parents and teachers from their primary task: the provision of an *individual* program to develop and enhance the communication skills of each hearing-impaired child.

Public school systems appear to be recognizing the heterogeneity of the hearing-impaired population by offering "two-track" programs employing both oral and total communication methods, while several systems have added cued speech as a third alternative. This development reflects a growing realization that the methods employed in education are but a means to an end—the development of communication skills—and that children will differ with respect to their ability to process incoming information and express their ideas. Quigley and Kretschmer (1982) stated that the topic of methodology involved two issues: language (American Sign Language or English) and form of communication (oral or manual). Various combinations of these language systems and communication forms define the methods curently used to educate hearing-impaired children.

The Auditory Approach

With the development of wearable hearing aids in the 1940s, a few audiologists and educators initiated an aggressive exploration of the extent to which hearing-impaired children could utilize audition. The unisensory approach, also referred to as the auditory approach or acoupedics (Pollack, 1970), is a habilitative procedure emphasizing the development of speech and language skills through the use of residual hearing.

Early detection and fitting of amplification enables the hearing-impaired child to take advantage of critical early years to develop communication skills. Both the parent and child are included in individual therapy sessions, in which the clinician demonstrates techniques to stimulate speech and language and to integrate hearing into the child's total environment. The parent is then expected to reinforce these skills with the child between sessions. The once-a-week sessions emphasize that it is the parent's use of daily routines for language experiences, not the therapy sessions, which are responsible for the development of communication skills. Formal speechreading is not taught, and the use of vision by the child is discouraged in an effort to develop the impaired modality to the fullest extent. Placement of the child in hearing nurseries and school settings provides normal role models and an enriched linguistic environment.

In answering critics of this method, professionals explain that the hearing loss is not being denied—the program attempts to remediate the effects of the hearing impairment through carefully planned, sequential steps—but, rather, habilitation seeks to help the child reach maximum potential through the development of speech and language competence.

The Multisensory Approach

The oral or multisensory approach employs several sensory modes simultaneously in providing language input to the hearing-impaired child.

Distinguishing between oral and auditory approaches is sometimes difficult because the terms "aural-oral" and "auditory-oral" are used by professionals to describe either of these two methods. Basically, the difference lies in the use of the auditory mode as the primary input for speech and language.

Like all approaches to educating hearing-impaired children, the oral approach stresses early detection, appropriate amplification, and parent involvement as important factors in the habilitation process. Unlike the auditory approach, the oral child learns speech skills and language concepts in large measure through a bimodal presentation: vision and audition, although exercises may be devised that emphasize speech reading or auditory training. The visual mode is assumed to be the prominent sense utilized by the child, although it may be augmented by audition and taction.

Educational programming also distinguishes the multisensory and unisensory approaches. While the oral infant is usually placed in a parent/infant program and seen on a weekly basis for individual therapy, the preschooler is usually educated in a special class for the hearing impaired (although parents are encouraged to integrate the child in a hearing nursery on a part-time basis). Thus, primary placement is in a special class rather than a normal-hearing setting.

Cued Speech

Cued speech is a visual-oral system designed to facilitate language development in hearing-impaired children by eliminating the ambiguities of speechreading. Devised by Orin Cornett (1967), it is a system of 8 hand configurations which represent the 25 English consonants, and 4 hand positions which represent 2-4 vowels each. The hand cues supplement information received through lipreading—that is, the child must continue to rely on both hand and speech cues for complete information. No single phoneme may be identified by hand cue alone, but must be "read" in conjunction with lip movements. For example, the sounds /p/, /b/, and /m/ are each represented by a different hand configuration which serves to distinguish the sounds. However, the hand configuration representing /p/ also represents /d/ and /zh/, making it impossible for the child to determine which of the three phonemes is being presented without also using speechreading. Cornett hypothesized that this system would enable the hearing impaired to learn language like a hearing child, free from ambiguity, yet through a visual rather than an auditory mode.

Cued speech is not widely employed in educational programs, but is gaining acceptance as a third alternative to oral and total communication programs.

Total Communication

Although manual communication is used by many deaf adults, it is rarely employed in educational settings with hearing-impaired children. The term "total communication" (also the "combined" or "simultaneous method") refers to programs which incorporate manual communication, (sign language and finger spelling), speech, auditory training, and amplification in an attempt to develop both verbal and manual abilities in hearing-impaired students. Supporters of this method believe that the addition of signs to the visual and auditory speech modes assists in overcoming the confusions which ensue from reliance upon speechreading and residual hearing.

One of the most serious problems faced by the proponents of total communication was the difference in linguistic structure between signed and written and spoken English—the language issue that Quigley and Kretschmer spoke of. Educators expressed concern over the ability of young hearing-impaired children to acquire fluency in English structure when presented with a manual language whose word order did not closely parallel that of English. As a result, several sign systems were created which attempted to accurately represent the syntactic structure of English (Bornstein, 1973).

Seeing Essential English (SEE 1) and Signing Exact English (SEE 2) are two manual systems which employ conventional English word order and utilize a combination of American Sign Language and invented signs to represent the English language. Each system has devised its own rules regarding the representation of spoken/written English in signs, and they differ slightly—SEE 2 using a greater number of traditional signs and fewer affixes than SEE 1. Signed English is a system originally created for use in the preschool at Gallaudet, and employs ASL signs with 14 additional signs for representing some of the English inflectional markers. Signs for pronouns, some auxilliaries, and subject-verb agreement have been devised, and as with the other two systems, English word order is followed.

In recent years many school systems which formerly offered only an oral method of instruction have added total communication as a second option. A study by Jordan, Gustason, and Rosen (1976) examined current communication trends in programs for the deaf and found that 64% were using total communication.

Educational Programming: Methodological Issues

All professionals concerned with hearing-impaired children face the selection of the appropriate communication method for education. Thus far, few efforts have been directed toward objectifying this decision and lessening the emotions generally involved in choosing a communication method.

Marion Downs (1972) attempted to objectify decisions regarding communication methods and to recommend habilitative programs based upon individual children's profiles. The Deafness Management Quotient (DMQ) examined factors believed to be predictors of a child's success in an oral program: severity of hearing loss, the integrity of the central nervous system, intellectual factors, family support, and socio-economic status. A 100-point scale was devised on which the child was rated with respect to each element, and the scores totaled. A sum of 81 or greater signified the likelihood of achievement in an oral program. While the DMQ has not been adopted by institutions across the United States, it points out that many factors which relate to both the child and family are important in successfully habilitating hearing losses. The development of similar guidelines and the assessment of other significant components such as preferred learning mode may enable the professional to determine earlier and more accurately the appropriate communication method.

Downs (Northern & Downs, 1974) suggested four priorities with respect to communication methodology which were pertinent to the development of individual programs for hearing-impaired children. It is essential that communities establish programs offering families of hearing-impaired children options regarding communication method, in order to ensure that the individual needs of the child are met. Another priority that Downs noted is the importance of developing assessment tools to evaluate a child's progress and objectify possible program changes in method or any other aspect. Downs also stated that audiologists should be familiar with different teaching methodologies to facilitate accurate counseling of parents. A fourth priority was the establishment of total communication programs at the preschool and infant levels of training. This last component is critical and is recognized by proponents of all methods as a vital factor in the success of any habilitation program.

The choice of a communication methodology for educating the hearing-impaired child is an important decision to be resolved by parents and professionals. The selection of any method influences the child's acquisition of communication skills, specifically the achievement of written and spoken/signed English, and has significant implications for the extent to which the child will be integrated into the mainstream of the "hearing" world. Efforts to verify one method over others arise from philosophies that fail to view the hearing-impaired population as a heterogeneous one, comprised of people who possess diverse skills and abilities.

Investigations of the hearing population have concluded that individuals have different learning styles. One might speculate that while some hearing-impaired individuals learn through a combinatioin of two or more modes, others best utilize a single channel for input. Certainly exploration of the learning process and the hearing impaired could enable professionals to assist parents in taking advantage of the methodological options available and selecting an appropriate one for each child.

Assessment

Accurate assessment is essential in planning individual programs designed to facilitate the development of academic and communication skills in an effective habilitative program. Public Law 94-142 specifies that evaluation procedures and objective criteria be used to determine that short-term goals are met (Dublinske, 1978). In planning effective programs for hearing-impaired children, it is important to determine the child's current level of achievement. The teacher/clinician can then build upon the child's previous skills, rather than attempt to teach a skill for which the child has no foundation. Evaluation procedures should also indicate future skills the child must acquire to ensure that teaching is an orderly, efficient process. This is especially important in a school district program where the child is changing teachers yearly. Assessment also assists the professional in determining the rate at which a child learns. This is not emphasized in the literature on the habilitation of the hearing impaired, but is an important consideration in programming instruction. Evaluations that indicate a slow rate of progress should motivate the clinician to examine the habilitation program. Ideally, the results of evaluations should provide educators with information helpful in the planning of individual educational programs and in the placement of children in appropriate learning environments.

However, the objective evaluation of hearing-impaired children also presents some specific problems for the teacher, educational psychologist, or other examiner who is evaluating the student. Few tests available today have been standardized on the hearing-impaired population; yet, out of necessity, these tools must be used with the hearing-impaired child. Some of the tests, however, may not be sensitive to the abilities, attitudes, or inclinations of the deaf (Garrison, 1979; Levine, 1971). Common problems in the administration of tests to hearing-impaired children have been identified by Rudner (1978). In examining tests which were standardized on the general population, Rudner found that some of the tests failed to evaluate items in the hearing-impaired curriculum, and the score a child received on an evaluation was not an accurate reflection of the knowledge acquired. Rudner also found that grade-equivalent scores could be meaningless and difficult to interpret for children in ungraded classrooms. In addition, other investigators noted that a larger variance characterized the scores of hearing-impaired as compared to hearing students (Anderson & Sisco, 1977). With respect to item appropriateness and test construction, reliability was usually lower for hearing-impaired students than for their hearing counterparts, thus increasing the measurement error of the scores. The use of certain syntactic structures and vocabulary items on evaluations has also placed the hearing-impaired child at a disadvantage when compared to hearing peers (McKee & Hausknecht, 1980). As a result of these problems, many assessment procedures fail to provide information necessary to construct an effective learning sequence for the hearing-impaired child.

Subjective teacher assessments are often used to evaluate students' academic performance. Despite the apparent accuracy of teacher judgments, however, rating scales are subjective and fail to provide information on the specific academic level at which students are functioning.

Educators have attempted to modify assessment tools standardized on the hearing population by adapting test procedures to accommodate the special needs of the deaf and by developing norms with hearing-impaired subjects. Efforts to remediate some of the problems encountered in assessing the deaf have resulted in the standardization of the WISC-R (Anderson & Sisco, 1977) on deaf children and in the development of the Standard Achievement Test-Hearing Impaired Edition (SAT-HI) for achievement testing (Trybus & Karchmer, 1977).

In addition to an audiological evaluation, assessment batteries often include tests selected to evaluate skills in the following areas: psychological; academic achievement; annd communication skills including language and speech.

Psychological Assessment

The evaluation of intellectual functioning and cognitive development is one of the most difficult areas to assess with respect to the hearing-impaired child because of the "verbal bias" of many tests. The hearing-impaired child with limited verbal skills may be unable to demonstrate possessed abilities. To overcome this disadvantage, accurate assessment often requires the use of nonverbal or performance tests in addition to verbal evaluations to measure intellectual capacity and cognitive skills. The following tests are frequently used with hearing-impaired children:

Columbia Mental Maturity Scale (CMMS)
Goodenough Draw-A-Man Test
Leiter International Performance Scale

McCarthy Scales of Children's Abilities (MSCA)
Nebraska Test of Learning Aptitude
Stanford-Binet Intelligence Scale
Wechsler Intelligence Scale for Children (WISC)
Wechsler Preschool and Primary Scale of Intelligence (WPPSI)

In addition, other assessment instruments may be used with young hearing-impaired infants:

Bayley Scales of Infant Development (BSID)
Cattell Infant Intelligence Scale
Denver Developmental Screening Test (DDST)
Gesell Developmental Schedules
Griffiths Mental Development Scale for Testing Babies from Birth to Two Years.
Minnesota Preschool Scale (MPS)
Ordinal Scales of Psychological Development

Critiques of these instruments and information on their use with hearing-impaired children can be found elsewhere (Educational Testing Service, 1974; Hasenstab & Horner, 1982); however, a few general remarks about psychological testing are pertinent.

Both verbal and nonverbal scores provide useful information for the clinician, and many of the above tools break down the full-scale quotient into verbal and performance components. Even when administering "nonverbal" tests, however, the examiner must be cautious about the verbal content of the instructions, which can influence scores. The use of two performance tests is recommended to assure accurate testing. Verbal scores may also be useful for assessment of a hearing-impaired child's skills, especially if one is considering mainstreaming a student. Verbal measures tend to be a better indicator of academic functioning than performance scores, and the results of verbal intelligence tests may provide information on the ability of the student to use verbal concepts, an important skill for successful integration.

Academic Achievement

The need to monitor carefully the level of educational achievement is emphasized by the poor academic performance of hearing-impaired students reported previously in this chapter. Academic assessment is usually performed by the teacher of the hearing impaired, resource room teacher, or regular classroom teacher, and includes formal assessment tools as well as informal observation. Both achievement tests and diagnostic tests are employed. The California Achievement Test (CAT), Wide Range Achievement Test (WRAT), and Stanford Achievement Test (SAT) evaluate the student's performance in a number of academic areas including reading, spelling, mathematics, social studies, and science. Scores are norm-referenced and reported as grade equivalent and/or percentile scores. The CAT, WRAT, and SAT have been normed on hearing populations and enable the professional to compare the performance of the hearing impaired to the hearing students. The Hearing-Impaired Edition of the Standford Achievement Test (SAT-HI) allows the teacher to compare the performance of hearing-impaired students to each other as well as to hearing peers. However, while comparisons to hearing-impaired norms may be appropriate for one child, the child who is mainstreamed into a regular classroom should test favorably with normally hearing children if integration is to be successful. In addition, the administration of the test should occur in the regular classroom under conditions similar to that during a normal school day.

Professionals are cautioned against frequent testing because of the large variation in the scores of hearing-impaired children. Small changes in scores may in fact be no larger than the standard error of measure. Achievement tests are designed only to give a general estimation of a student's level of performance. As with psychological testing, an item-by-item analysis of the student's test often yields information that more accurately describes the student's strengths and weaknesses, and is more useful in planning teaching strategies to remediate deficits than an overall score.

For a more in-depth analysis of the student's academic performance in specific areas such as reading, math, and spelling, diagnostic tests are employed in addition to a general achievement test battery. The Peabody Individual Achievement Test (PIAT), Key Math, Woodcock-Johnson, Gates-McGinitie, and Metropolitan Readiness tests are examples of frequently employed diagnostic evaluations.

Communication Skills Assessment

The foundation of any habilitation program for the hearing impaired is the development of receptive and expressive communication skills, specifically the development of written and spoken/signed English. Although few assessment tools have been designed to evaluate faults typical of the hearing-impaired population, knowledge of these communication difficulties and normal language development enable the clinician to choose appropriate instruments for evaluation.

Observation, whether informally noted or charted on formal scales, becomes very important in evaluating the communication abilities of hearing-impaired children. Parental reports may also assist the clinician in determining the type of formal testing to be pursued.

Speech Assessment

Information on the ability of the hearing-impaired child to correctly produce speech with reference not only to normally hearing peers but also to common speech errors among the hearing impaired would appear to be an important consideration in selecting an evaluation tool. Few commercially available evaluations formally assess these features, however. Oftentimes, sounds are evaluated only in the context of words and not in babbled syllables. This is an important distinction for the hearing-impaired child who may be able to correctly articulate a sound in syllables but is experiencing difficulty in transferring phonemes to meaningful contexts. For the child with low verbal abilities, the use of unfamiliar vocabulary items may influence the accuracy of the evaluation. In addition, most tests fail to assess specific prosodic features such as breath control, stress, and intonation—features which are produced with difficulty by many deaf individuals and which serve as the foundation for the development of articulation skills. The Phonetic Level and Phonological Level Evaluations which accompany the Ling Speech Program were designed to be used within the context of a comprehensive speech program for the hearing-impaired child. Speech is assessed through direct imitation at the phonetic level and in a spontaneous speech sample at the phonological level. Prosodic features are also evaluated. No norms have been established for the test; however, the evaluation does clearly delineate the child's level of performance and outlines the next speech goals. For the child with adequate language ability, the following articulation tests may prove useful in assessment:

> *Deep Test of Articulation*
> *Developmental Articulation Test*
> *Fisher-Logemann Test of Articulation Competence*
> *Goldman-Fristoe Test of Articulation (GFTA)*
> *Templin-Darley Tests of Articulation (TDTA)*

Language Assessment

Language provides the foundation upon which the child develops written, spoken, and signed English, yet, as with other areas of assessment, few standardized language tests evaluate the problems typically experienced by the hearing impaired in learning language.

The use of both formal standardized tests and language sampling procedures is recommended for an accurate evaluation of linguistic competence. The choice of an evaluation instrument is important because most assessment tools tend to focus on one aspect of language, expressive or receptive skills for example, or may evaluate primarily one language component, usually vocabulary or syntax. Few formal tests evaluate semantic and pragmatic components. Kretschmer and Kretschmer (1978) present an excellent review of language-assessment tools employed with the hearing impaired. Results obtained from any assessment are influenced by the format of the test. A variety of formats are used to evaluate language: elicited imitation as employed in the expressive portion of the Northwestern Syntax Screening Test (NSST) and the Elicited Language Inventory (ELI); demonstration tasks which appear in several tests from the Reynell Language Developmental Tasks and the Preschool Language Scale; picture or object identification utilized in the Peabody Picture Vocabulary Test (PPVT); and grammatical judgment exemplified in the Test of Syntactic Abilities (TSA).

Kretschmer and Kretschmer caution readers about interpreting results from any test without considering the influence of the interaction between the examiner, the child, and the test format. Performance on the ELI or the NSST, for example, may be influenced by the child's ability to be "imitative," the rate of presentation by the examiner, and the length of the stimulus material. In using a demonstration task or object manipulation format, the examiner is cautioned to be aware of offering situational cues to the child, and to look for the child's preference for certain objects or activities. Presentation rate, guessing, and the use of appropriate foils for test items are important issues for consideration with respect to picture-identification tasks. Tests utilizing grammatical judgment formats are appropriate for older and linguistically more sophisticated children.

Several assessment tools have been designed recently for use with the hearing-impaired child and are useful additions to traditional language evaluation batteries. The Test of Syntactic Abilities (Steinkamp & Quigley, 1976) is designed to measure the syntactic competencies of the hearing impaired through the use of a grammatical judgment format. The TSA evaluates eight aspects of English syntax and has been normed on hearing-impaired children ages 10-18. Because it is a written evaluation, it is only useful for older children. The battery consists of a Screening Test and Diagnostic Battery to provide in-depth information on students' strengths and weaknesses in specific syntactic structures; however, because the tests uses a multiple-choice format, it only assesses receptive abilities and not the spontaneous productions of the child. Another test recently developed to evaluate the syntactic structures of hearing-impaired children is the Grammatical Analysis of Elicited Language (GAEL). In a series of three tests, the GAEL evaluates language at the presentence, simple sentence, and complex sentence levels, utilizing toys, games, and stories through spontaneous production and elicited imitation. Each test has been normed on hearing-impaired and normal-hearing children, and information on future language goals as well as current level of functioning is easily available.

Evaluating the communication skills of young hearing-impaired infants is especially challenging. Observation of the child in informal activities is even more important than with older children because formal testing procedures often do not reflect the infant's best performance. Thus, assessment procedures often include interviews and observational scales. The Receptive-Expressive Emergent Language Scale (REEL) is an example of an assessment tool that employs parent interviews to elicit information on linguistic performance. Obviously, the accuracy of this assessment relies on the parents' observational skills and may only provide the clinician with a general idea of the child's level of functioning. From that point, the clinician may wish to pursue formal testing and language sampling. However, from the interview the clinician might also gain useful insights into the parent's perceptions of their child, which is also valuable information in planning appropriate programs for family intervention.

Several scales have also been designed that examine not only language but other areas of development as well. No formal evaluation procedures are usually defined; rather, the clinician devises activities that assess the skill and determines if the competency has been achieved. Ling (1977) and Moog and Geers (1975) have proposed two such methods of assessment. Ling's Schedules of Development evaluates specific auditory, speech, language, and communication skills. Behaviors are listed in the order of difficulty and the clinician or parent dates the achievement of each skill. The Scales of Early Communication Skills for Hearing Impaired Children (Moog & Geers, 1975) examines the child's performance in terms of language and nonverbal communication skills. Both receptive and expressive behaviors are rated, and criteria are suggested for judgment. The Development Assessment Schema (Northcott, 1977) evaluates expressive and receptive speech and language, gross and fine motor, personal-social, perceptuo-cognitive, self-help, and auditory skills. Age norms for hearing children are listed for each behavior, and the clinician notes accomplishment of the behaviors. Each of these scales is useful for both parents and professionals in providing a general estimate of the child's performance, and as a general guide for designing long-range teaching objectives.

Language Sampling

Sampling the spontaneous language production of hearing-impaired children enables the professional to determine language competency with respect to semantic and pragmatic features as well as syntactic abilities. Analysis of language samples augments information received from formal tests and also points out areas the professional may want to probe further through the use of a specific evaluation instrument. For example, a clinician concerned about the use of question forms by a hearing-impaired child may probe further by administering the Test of Syntactic Abilities or by contriving natural situations and recording the child's spontaneous conversation. The use of conversation, objects, and pictures in eliciting a sample demonstrates the child's facility in using language to convey information. Observation of the child's use of language with peers and parents, and written samples provide added information useful in assessing language competence in different communication situations.

Procedures for analyzing the spontaneous language of hearing-impaired children have been adapted from protocols used with the language-impaired population, such as those developed by Lee (1974), Tyack and Gottsleben (1974), and by Crystal, Fletcher, and Garman (1976). The above sampling procedures focus on syntactic development and are limited in their ability to define pragmatic and semantic difficulties. The Developmental Sentence Analysis (Lee, 1974) is actually composed of two analyses, the Developmental Sentence Types and the Developmental Sentence Scoring, which allow the professional to analyze language at the presentence and sentence levels. The analysis developed by Tyack and Gottsleben is similar in its emphasis on syntax; however, it is developmentally organized and enables the clinician to more easily establish goals for the child's language program. The procedure developed by Crystal and associates describes derivations from normal patterns in addition to a basic syntactic analysis. Such descriptions are especially useful in planning remediation for hearing-impaired children. However, one major drawback of each of these procedures is the failure to look at semantic and pragmatic aspects of language. Scroggs (1977) employed the eight semantic functions described by Brown (1973) in analyzing the language of hearing-impaired adolescents who showed significant language delay and found the analysis useful in summarizing the semantic functions employed by the students. A more formal analysis was developed by Bloom and Lahey (1978) and examines syntax (form) as an outgrowth of semantics (content) and pragmatics (function). Like most other procedures, however, it fails to list the deviations from normal development. An analysis by Kretschmer and Kretschmer (1978) attempts to describe both language delays and differences, semantic content, syntax, communication competence, and deviations from normal development of semantics, syntax, and pragmatics.

No one sampling procedure may be appropriate for all children or provide the teacher with the necessary information to design a language program. Sampling must be recognized as an ongoing process, one in which results can differ according to the setting and stimuli provided. As in formal language and speech tests, it is essential that the clinician recognize the purpose of the evaluation and choose a sampling instrument that will assess the competencies in question.

Educational Programming: The Multidisciplinary Team Approach

Accurate assessment requires that data be collected from multiple sources, including the use of standard psychological and achievement tests, results from language and speech evaluations, and observational reports. A team approach is recommended when programming instructional objectives. The team should include a teacher of the hearing-impaired, educational psychologist, speech-language pathologist, audiologist, regular classroom teacher, and if appropriate, parents, and other interested professionals. In this way information on the child's performance in a number of different situations and on a variety of tasks is reviewed. For example, the informal observations of the teacher may illustrate some of the results found during testing, while, at the same time, formal assessment can pinpoint behaviors noted by other professionals and family.

Another important component in assessment is knowledge by the examiner of hearing-impaired children and the impact of hearing loss on the development of academic and communication skills. The examiner's ability to communicate with the child, to select an appropriate test battery, and to analyze test results is essential.

No assessment tool is infallible; however, by using several test instruments and evaluating input from different sources and situations, the probability of error is reduced, and the results useful in developing goals for remediation.

Placement Options

Programming for the Hearing-Impaired Infant

One of the most universally accepted trends in the education of hearing-impaired children has been the establishment of early intervention programs for parents and infants. Regardless of differences in communication methodology, models of speech and language development, and almost every other aspect of habilitation, professionals recognize the critical importance of early intervention in developing the communication skills of the infant and in helping the parents to become effective language facilitators.

During the first year of life, the burden of communication rests with the parent. This does not imply that the child lacks communicative ability, because we know that through smiles, squeals, and vocalizations the child "talks" with family and friends. However, it is the parent who weaves these behaviors—some intentional and others occurring spontaneously—into a dialogue created with the young baby. Through these early "conversations," the child learns about the pragmatic features of conversation such as turntaking, and, later, semantic and syntactic aspects of language. The parents efforts are usually rewarded at a year by the utterance of the first word as verbal behaviors emerge. At this point, the child becomes increasingly active in the conversation and begins to assume part of the burden of dialogue. The role of the parent in early language learning is essential. The reinforcement of early attempts by the infant to communicate, the establishment of parent-child turn-taking behaviors, and the linguistic input of the parent all contribute to the child's development of communication competence. Most important is the quality of interaction between the parent and young child. It is this quality that lays the foundation upon which the child learns to converse with others.

The parent of the hearing-impaired child is confronted with a child who fails to respond to parental attempts to converse, or who responds inconsistently. Prior to intervention, this frustration and the anxiety over the possibility of a hearing loss may result in the breakdown of communication between parent and child. For the family with a child whose loss is undiagnosed until 18 months or 2 years, there is often a complete disruption in interaction.

The goals of early intervention are to establish a positive interaction between parent and child that serves as a basis for developing speech and language. As such, programs encompass the following principles:

1. Early detection of hearing loss followed by appropriate fitting of amplification and audiological management;

2. The provision of support services to the parent, including emotional support for understanding and coping with the hearing loss; the provision of information to understand the ramifications of a hearing impairment; and demonstration of techniques to facilitate language learning, speech training, and auditory skill development;

3. An individualized therapeutic program designed to develop not only communication needs of the child, but also needs in other areas as necessary;

4. The use of an experiential approach to language learning.

In contrast to most other habilitative procedures, the parent—not the child—is the primary target of early intervention programs. Like the parent of a hearing child, the parent of a hearing-impaired child is the most influential person in the child's environment. By focusing on the parent, the program offers emotional support and seeks to give the parent the knowledge needed to understand the hearing loss and its implications for the educational, social, and emotional development of the child. Guidance and counseling are the first critical needs of any parent of an exceptional child. Through individual sessions as well as group meetings, parents learn to share and discuss their feelings and experiences. The clinician seeks to demonstrate to the parent techniques for facilitating the development of language, auditory, and speech skills. Through demonstrations in structured and unstructured activities, and observation of the parent and child, the clinician is able to help the parent modify speaking habits. The parent learns to utilize daily activities such as bathing and washing clothes to stimulate communication with the infant.

The parent is seen as a partner in the education process, and this role is reinforced in several ways. Sessions usually are scheduled once a week to emphasize the importance of the home environment, and not the therapeutic sessions. Parents are encouraged to observe their child and report observations to the clinician, who then devises an individual program based upon the needs of the family as a group. One of the major objectives of a parent/infant program is the development of independence and confidence within the parent. Parents learn about audiograms, hearing aids, as well as speech and language development. This knowledge serves as a foundation for building realistic expectations for the child and for formulating educational goals. Knowledge of the child's rights and parents' responsibilities under Public Law 94-142 enables parents to become effective advocates for their school-aged child, just as they learned to become effective communicators with their infant.

Programming for the School-aged Hearing-Impaired Child

Not only the young infant has benefited from innovations responding to the mandates of PL94-142. The school-aged hearing-impaired child has available a variety of eductional programs which offer the opportunity to be instructed with hearing peers in a variety of placements.

Three models of programming are used by educators, and order program alternatives along a continuum from "most restrictive" to "least restrictive" (Deno, 1970; Dunn, 1973; Reynolds, 1962). Although the three models differ in the number of programs specified for mainstreaming handicapped children, the similarities between the models emphasize concepts accepted in the education of all handicapped children, including the hearing-impaired student. The number of placement options offered in each model emphasizes the desire to provide programming for hearing-impaired children whose skills and abilities differ greatly and to recognize the variations in these students.

Each model also recognizes the importance of offering the student the opportunity to be educated with normal-hearing peers whenever possible, yet provide the necessary support to fulfill academic goals.

Hein and Bishop (1979) provide an excellent summary of program options. Placement in a regular classroom, either with or without the services of a special educator, is the most integrated environment, designed for the student who is functioning on grade level in core academic subjects. These students tend to be the less severely involved (although this does not necessarily imply the less severe hearing losses). The itinerant may provide tutorial services for the student for a portion of the day (usually not more than one hour) or may serve as a consultant to the regular classroom teacher. The resource room provides assistance for the student who is able to be mainstreamed for some academic subjects, but who requires help by a special teacher for 2-4 hours a day. The student in a resource room usually performs at grade level for some subjects, but below hearing peers for others. However, individual communciation skills are such that the student is able to perform for part of the day in regular classrooms. The student requiring full-time services of a special teacher is usually placed in a self-contained classroom, which may be in a regular school or in a special day school. These more severely involved students are functioning two or more grades behind hearing peers, so integration in a regular classroom for academic subjects would fail to meet their educational goals. Instruction in all academic subjects is by a teacher of the hearing-impaired, or other special education personnel, and accompanied by integration for nonacademic subjects like art, physical education, and lunch, if possible. The most restrictive educational setting is a residential/hospital facility or home-bound instruction.

Although the integration of hearing-impaired children with other normal hearing individuals is a concept educators have adopted and incorporated into school programs, especially during the last decade, some controversy exists regarding mainstreaming as a goal, or as a means by which educational goals are achieved. Hein and Bishop (1979) state the importance of viewing mainstreaming as a means to the goal of educating hearing-impaired children in an environment that allows them the opportunity to develop to their fullest potential. For some children, this goal is best met by integration in a regular classroom, while for others integration on a part-time basis or placement in a self-contained classroom is most appropriate.

Summary

As a result of federal legislation, professionals working with hearing-impaired children have recognized the importance of offering learning environments best suited to meet the needs of the students. The importance of assessment in determining performance level and designing programs for hearing-impaired children was emphasized in the provisions of Public Law 94-142, and educators have responded by designing assessment tools to measure specific concerns related to educating the hearing impaired. The establishment of parent/infant programs has assisted parents in becoming active participants in educational decision making and in providing the early language-learning environment important for the development of speech and language. Yet, professionals working with the hearing impaired realize a continuing need to design effective programs to develop the communication skills necessary for the hearing impaired to become productive members of society.

References

Anderson, R., & Sisco, F. *Standardization of the WISC-R Performance Scale for deaf children.* Series T, Number 1, Washington, DC: Gallaudet College, Office of Demographic Studies, 1977.

Blackwell, P.M., Engen, E., Fischgrund, J.E., & Zarcadoolas C. Sentences and other systems. Washington, DC: Alexander Graham Bell Association for the Deaf, 1978.

Bloom, L., & Lahey, M. *Language development and language disorders.* New York: John Wiley, 1978.

Bornstein, H. A description of some current sign systems designed to represent English. *American Annals of the Deaf,* 1973, *118,* 454-463.

Brown, R. *A first language: The early stages.* Cambridge, MA: Harvard University Press, 1973.

Calvert, D.R., & Silverman, S.R. *Speech and deafness.* Washington, DC: The Alexander Graham Bell Association for the Deaf, 1975.

Clarke School for the Deaf. *Speech development: Curriculum evaluation and Development Program.* Northampton, MA: Clarke School for the Deaf, 1971.

Cornett, O. Cued Speech. *American Annals of the Deaf,* 1967, *112,* 3-13.

Crystal, D., Fletcher, P., & Garman, M. *The grammatical analysis of language disability: A procedure for assessment and remediation.* New York: Elsevier-North Holland, 1976.

Deno, E. Special education as developmental capital. *Exceptional Children,* 1970, *37,* 229-397.

Downs, M. Basis for choosing the appropriate habilitation program. Paper presented at the American Speech and Hearing Convention, San Francisco, November, 1972.

Dublinske, S. PL 94-142: Developing the individualized education program (IEP). *Asha,* 1978, *20,* 380-397.

Dunn, L. (Ed.) *Exceptional children in the public schools: Special education in transition* (2nd ed.). New York: Holt, Rinehart & Winston, 1973.

Educational Testing Service. Tests for the deaf and hearing impaired. *Test Collection.* Princeton, NJ: 1974.

Fitzgerald, E. *Straight language for the deaf.* Washington, DC: The Alexander Graham Bell Association for the Deaf, 1949.

Garrison, W. Examinations, examiners and their interaction. *The Volta Review,* 1979, *81,* 431-435.

Geers, A., & Moog, J. Syntactic maturity of spontaneous speech and elicited imitations of hearing-impaired children. *Journal of Speech and Hearing Disorders,* 1978, *43,* 380-391.

Groht, M. *National language for deaf children.* Washington, DC: The Alexander Graham Bell Association for the Deaf, 1958.

Hasenstab, M.S., & Horner J.S. *Comprehensive intervention with hearing-impaired infants and preschool children.* Rockville, Maryland: Aspen Systems, 1982.

Haycock, G.S. *The teaching of speech.* Washington, DC: The Alexander Graham Bell Association for the Deaf, 1933.

Hein, R., & Bishop, M. Models and processes of mainstreaming. In M. Bishop, (Ed.), *Mainstreaming.* Washington, DC: Alexander Graham Bell Association for the Deaf, 1979.

Jordan, I.K., Gustason, G., & Rosen, R. Current communication trends at programs for the deaf. *American Annals of the Deaf,* 1976, *121,* 527-796.

Kretschmer, R. The writing ability of hearing-impaired and normally hearing children: Findings and applications. Paper presented at the Annual Meeting of the Alexander Graham Bell Association for the Deaf, Toronto, 1982.

Kretschmer, R., & Kretschmer, L. *Language development and intervention with the hearing impaired.* Baltimore: University Park Press, 1978.

Lee, L. *Developmental sentence analysis.* Evanston, ILL: Northwestern University Press, 1974.

Levine, E. Mental assessment of the deaf child. *The Volta Review,* 1971, *73,* 80-119.

Ling, A.H. *Schedules of development.* Washington, DC: The Alexander Graham Bell Association for the Deaf, 1977.

Ling, D. *Speech and the hearing-impaired child: Theory and practice.* Washington, DC: The Alexander Graham Bell Association for the Deaf, 1975.

Ling, D., Leckie, D., Pollack, D., Simser, J., & Smith, A. Syllable reception by hearing-impaired children trained from infancy in auditory-oral programs. *The Volta Review,* 1981, *83,* 451-457.

McKee, B., & Hausknecht, M. Classroom assessment techniques for hearing impaired students: A literature review. *Directions: Assessment of Hearing Impaired Youth,* 1980, *1,* 9-15.

Milne, M., & Ling, D. The development of speech in hearing-impaired children. In F. Bess, B. Freeman, & J. Sinclair, (Eds.), *Amplification in education.* Washington, DC: Alexander Graham Bell Association for the Deaf, 1981.

Moog, J., & Geers, A. *Scales of early communication skills for hearing impaired children.* St. Louis: Central Institute for the Deaf, 1975.

Nicholls, G. *Cued speech and the reception of spoken language.* Unpublished Masters thesis, McGill University, 1979.

Northcott, W. (Ed.) *Curriculum guide—hearing-impaired children—birth to three years—and their parents.* Washington, DC: Alexander Graham Bell Association for the Deaf, 1977.

Northern J.L., & Downs, M.P. *Hearing in children.* Baltimore: Williams & Wilkins, 1974.

Pollack D. *Educational audiology for the limited hearing infant.* Springfield, ILL: Charles C. Thomas, 1970.

Quigley, S., Power, D., & Steinkamp, M. The language structure of deaf children. *The Volta Review,* 1977, *79,* 73-84.

Quigley, S.P., & Kretschmer, R.E. *The education of deaf children.* Baltimore: University Park Press, 1982.

Rawlings, B.W., & Trybus, R.J. Personnel, facilities and services available in schools and classes for hearing impaired children in the United States. *American Annals of the Deaf,* 1978, *123,* 99-114.

Reynolds, M. A framework for considering some issues on special education. *Exceptional Children,* 1962, *28,* 367-370.

Rowe, L. The speech model. *The Volta Review,* 1974, *72,* 107-112.

Rudner, L. Using standard tests with the hearing impaired: The problem of item bias. *The Volta Review,* 1978, *80,* 31-40.

Scroggs, C. Analyzing the language of hearing impaired children with severe language acquisition problems. *American Annals of the Deaf,* 1977, *122,* 403-406.

Speech Development-Curriculum Series 1971. Northampton, MA: Clarke School for the Deaf.

Steinkamp, M., & Quigley, S. Assessing deaf children's written language. *The Volta Review,* 1976, *78,* 10-18.

Trybus, R.J., & Karchmer, M.A. School achievement scores of hearing impaired children: National data on achievement status and growth patterns. *American Annals of the Deaf,* 1977, *122,* 62-69.

Tyack, D., & Gottsleben, R. *Language sampling, analysis and training: A handbook for teachers and clinicians.* Palo Alto, CA: Consulting Psychological Press, 1974.

Vernon, M., & Koh, S. Effects of early manual communication on the achievement of deaf children. *American Annals of the Deaf,* 1970, *115,* 527-536.

Freeman E. McConnell

Legislative Issues in the Habilitation of the Hearing-Impaired

Identifying Hearing Impaired Children

A first step in evaluating whether there are major unmet needs of hearing-impaired children in our society is to determine the adequacy of programs that purport to identify those in whom hearing sensitivity is less than that generally defined as within normal limits. The Committee on Identification Audiometry (Darley, 1961) recommended more than two decades ago that this ascertaining step, the discovery of a hearing impairment that results in setting apart an individual for further examination and monitoring, be referred to as "identification audiometry." It is a technique designed to separate in a simple, rapid, and inexpensive manner those individuals who have a hearing disorder from those with normal hearing. Bess and McConnell (1981) describe it as a "preventive measure that emphasizes early detection and prompt medical intervention and/or habilitation," and state that the objective in children is to "eliminate or minimize any hearing loss that could affect learning." The younger the child, the more serious are the barriers to learning, inasmuch as normal cognitive and language development in the infant is highly dependent upon an intact sensory system of hearing. In turn, the formal education process that for most children begins by age 5 or 6 years is predicated on an assumption that the child's language functioning is well established and commensurate with that of his or her peers. Even mild hearing loss is a deterring factor to learning in the classroom where imparting and receiving of information occur almost constantly through the auditory modality.

Status of Current Practice

The use of identification audiometry is not new. Its inception in selected locales is virtually coincident with the appearance of the earliest commercial pure-tone audiometers 40 or more years ago. In that interval of time the accumulated experience of professionals in the field has resulted in many advancements characterizing current practice in this area. A landmark study by Eagles, Wishik, Doerfler, Melnick, and Levine (1963) demonstrated the ineffectiveness of pure-tone audiometry for detecting the presence of middle ear disease. The development of electroacoustic impedance audiometry in subsequent years has enhanced our ability to determine the presence of middle ear disease in many instances where the hearing level, as determined by pure-tone audiometry, remains within normal limits. Bess and McConnell (1981) point out the importance of adapting procedures to one's goals in implementing identification programs. If the goal is to identify hearing loss, pure-tone audiometry is the test of choice; if the goal is to detect middle ear disease, electroacoustic impedance measures should be used. The two methods used in combination, of course, can yield important information that neither can do alone.

Hearing screening of children occurs most often in the nation's schools because they afford the easiest access to the largest number of children at any given time. The availability and comprehensiveness of these programs vary greatly from state to state, however. Citing data from a survey of state screening programs, the above authors show that fewer than half the 50 states have considered identification programs of sufficient importance to pass legislation requiring hearing screening in the schools. Furthermore, there is great variability in such factors as qualifications of personnel who conduct the programs, the age and grade level of the children screened, and the agencies responsible for the screening.

When we consider identification programs for neonates, infants, and preschoolers, those for school-age children appear almost advanced in comparison. Downs (1976) has cited figures from a National Academy of Science report indicating that only 3% of the children from 6 months to 11 years had had a screening hearing test at their primary health care source. The relative inaccessibility of infants and preschoolers, once they have left the hospital after the neonatal period, is of course one reason for the lack of uniform programs of hearing screening before school age. Programs that do exist are most usually conducted in well-baby clinics of local health departments, day-care centers, and Head Start programs, and consequently tend to be confined primarily to children from lower socioeconomic levels.

Although a satisfactory technique to permit hearing screening of all newborns is not yet established, the Joint Committee on Infant Hearing Screening (composed of members from the American Speech-Language-

Hearing Association, the American Academy of Pediatrics, and the American Academy of Ophthalmology and Otorhinolaryngology) recommends the high-risk register for congenital hearing loss. They believe it can increase the identification of hearing impairment at birth by as much as tenfold. The Joint Committee further commends the application of an arousal test during a state of sleep as a supplement to the high-risk register. They encourage field trials of other behavioral screening tests that satisfy the requirements set forth in their 1970 statement with respect to stimuli, response patterns, environmental factors, status at the time of testing, and behavior of observers (Mencher, 1977). Identification of infants in the newborn nursery who are at risk for hearing impairment includes the presence of one or more of the following:

> History of congenital hearing loss in the family;
>
> Rubella or other nonbacterial intrauterine fetal infection;
>
> Defects of ear, nose, or throat;
>
> Birthweight less than 1,500 grams; and
>
> Bilirubin level greater than 20 mg/100 ml serum.

Downs (1977) reported results from a 5-year high risk program supplemented by arousal testing conducted at the University of Colorado Medical Center. She obtained a yield of 1 in each 40 newborns identified to be in the high-risk category; the presence of hearing loss in these infants was confirmed in the period from birth to 8 months of age. She believes use of the High Risk Register, supplemented by arousal testing has gained acceptance as a valid means of accomplishing newborn hearing screening. The problem lies in how best to educate professional personnel and lawmakers so that a national commitment will prevail. Horton and Hanners (1977) have deplored the apathy characterizing members of the health professions, including a number of our own colleagues in audiology and speech pathology, concerning this matter. They state that more concern is focused on the problems of massive screening than on the subsequent problems encountered by hearing-impaired children who are not identified in the first year of life.

Needs

Identification audiometry has been described as the first step in implementation and provision of programs that will ensure all hearing-impaired children in a given state are afforded an opportunity to develop and learn in accordance with their native potential, despite the handicap of poor hearing. Yet a summary of state screening programs (Bess &

McConnell, 1981) shows that hearing screening of school-age children is required by legislation in only 21 of the 50 states. Because screening for diseases is a prerogative of the states rather than of the federal government, it will be necessary for concerned professionals in the health fields to mount campaigns in their various states to change the current situation. It could well become a nation-wide effort through coordination of the state speech-language-hearing associations to push for state-mandated programs.

Identification programs for newborns, infants, and preschoolers have fared poorly insofar as attention from state lawmakers is concerned. Only two states from the survey cited above reported screening of preschool children below kindergarten, and it was required in only one of those two. Newborn screening is not mandated by any state legislature, although Downs (1977) commends the approach made in the state of Maryland, where an 11-member Commission on Hereditary Disorders has been created to write rules and regulations governing all genetic disease programs in that state. Since 50% or more of all congenital hearing disorders are estimated to be hereditary, hearing loss would be included. Downs further points out that hearing loss compares very favorably with other diseases screened at birth, in that the yield in hearing screening is greater than that for most others on which data are available. For example, she cites figures supporting 1 in 1,000 for hearing loss compared with phenylketinuria (PKU) occurring once in 15,000 births, and for which 90% of all newborns in this country receive obligatory PKU screening. Hence, hearing loss should rank very high in priority among diseases that can be screened at birth. The demonstrated success with the High Risk Register, combined with arousal tests, speaks eloquently for stepping up the number of programs in existence.

Furthermore, the value of early identification in the first year of life with appropriate interventions has also been adequately demonstrated. The longer detection is delayed, the more serious are the ramifications for the individual child's language development, educational achievement, and ultimate vocational status. Identification programs for newborns are the best solution when and if planning for the appropriate medical and educational interventions is carried out following detection. At no other period during the preschool years does the accessibility of every child become more nearly possible, and state-mandated identification programs at that period in every child's life would greatly assist us to overcome the strategic gap between birth and the time when the child starts school. An important challenge for the future, then, is how we can best establish newborn hearing screening as a routine effort throughout our nation.

Early Views on Education of Hearing-Impaired Children

The right of every child to a free public education has long been a basic concept running parallel with the development of the public education system in the United States. In practice, however, it did not materialize easily for many of our nation's handicapped children. Hearing-impaired children have been no exception in this regard. For this reason, the passage of the Education of All Handicapped Children Act of 1975 was viewed as a major landmark in the realization of this goal. Those committed to providing adequate educational opportunity for hearing-impaired children face two critical challenges in the 1980s. The first of these is the successful implementation of the act throughout the nation's school systems; the second is the preservation of many of the important rights and protections provided for in the act that may be lost in an era of changing attitudes and priorities held by the federal government.

In this section, some of the earliest documented perceptions of society regarding the educability of the deaf, together with changes in attitudes and subsequent changes in opportunity that have come about up to the present time, are presented.

Slow Pace toward Enlightenment

References to the deaf prior to the 16th century are neither frequent nor detailed, but Aristotle in the pre-Christian era wrote, "Those born deaf all become speechless," thereby indicating recognition of some relation between early childhood deafness and muteness (DeLand, 1931). It is not clear if he did in fact recognize the causal nature of this relationship, however, and because deaf children were unable to speak or understand the speech of others, he believed them incapable of instruction. Hebrew law differentiated between those who were deaf and mute and those who were deaf only, or, in other words, between prelingual and postlingual deafness. The Talmud classified those in the former category with fools and children and denied them legal rights. Deaf mutes were similarly excluded by the Justinian Code from the rights and obligations of citizenship later, during the Roman period (6th centry A.D.). The first source of an enlightened attitude toward the intellectual capabilities of the prelingually deaf came from the writings of the Venerable Bede in the 7th century. He referred to the success of Bishop John of York in teaching a deaf and dumb young man to speak intelligibly.

The European continent then entered the period known as the Dark Ages, and several hundred years passed before any further recording of successful accomplishments in this area was made—or if so, has come to light. It was not until the late Renaissance (16th century) that a growing recognition that the deaf can indeed be taught may be discerned in the works of various writers describing the earliest methods of teaching. An Italian physician named Girolamo Cardano, referring to the work of Rudolphus Agricola in the Netherlands, set forth in the mid-16th century important principles which promised a more optimistic outlook for the deaf than any theretofore described. He wrote that it is possible "to place a deaf-mute in a position to hear by reading, and to speak by writing; for his memory leads him to understand, by reflection, that *bread*, as written, signifies the thing which is eaten" (DeLand, 1931). In essence, Cardano was proposing what would later be known as the association method, whereby a given written symbol and sets of symbols would be learned through presenting them in combination with objects representing them. Silverman (1970), who credits Cardano for his concept rejecting the widely held theory that the deaf were not capable of being educated, says Cardano's writings constitute what essentially was an educational Magna Carta for the deaf.

Other references to the ability of the deaf to learn came from Spain where Pedro Ponce de Leon (also in the 16th century) taught two deaf sons of a wealthy nobleman's family, and thus enabled the elder to acquire enough language to claim his birthright. In the 17th century, the earliest known text on articulation teaching was published in Madrid. Juan Pablo Bonet, the author of *The Method of Teaching Deaf Mutes to Speak*, published in 1620, displayed an unusual grasp of some of the intricacies of teaching speech and language to deaf children. He advocated the use of the manual language in connection with speech teaching. Dalgarno of Scotland published a manual alphabet in 1661, and in 1690 Amman, a physician in Amsterdam, published his famous *Surdus Loquens*, in which he described his method of teaching the deaf and dumb to talk and hear with their eyes. Following the appearance of this work, a new interest in lipreading was generated, particularly in Germany. These earliest efforts to teach the deaf, however, were aimed more at the deaf children of the aristocracy than the general populace. There was also great concern among the clerics of that time regarding the spirtual status of the deaf.

The 18th century marked the opening of the first public schools for the deaf, one in Germany and one in France, by two men of great vision, Samuel Heinicke and the Abbé de l'Epée, each committed to his convictions that deaf children must be provided the opportunity to become educated. The two men disagreed on method, however, and each vigorously defended his own. The Abbé de l'Epée had learned Spanish so that he could read Bonet's book which led him to adopt the sign language as the method for the school that he opened in Paris in 1775 for deaf children of all income levels. His school was operated as a state school as a result of financial support granted him by King Louis XVI. Heinicke was convinced that speech and speechreading should be stressed to the exclusion of signs in teaching deaf children. These differences in approach characterized the trends for educational programs in countries throughout the world, including the United States. The contributions made by these two great educators, however, are not dependent upon their differences but on their activism in demonstrating that deaf children can learn if afforded special instruction designed to meet their unique needs. This significant tenet was firmly established by the end of the 18th century as a result of their pioneering efforts. For a more detailed account of the historical background of educational treatment of hearing-impaired children, the reader may wish to consult the following references: DeLand (1931), Bender (1960), and Silverman (1970).

Development of Educational Programs in the United States

A few attempts were made in this country to organize educational programs for the deaf even prior to the colonies' struggle for independence, but none of these endured. Hartford, Connecticut, in 1817, became the site of the first permanent school. Much of the impetus for this school, the American Asylum for the Education and Instruction of the Deaf and Dumb (now the American School for the Deaf), was provided by Thomas Hopkins Gallaudet, a young divinity student. A group of influential New Englanders had sponsored his visit to Europe to learn about methods of instruction being used there to educate deaf children. When his efforts to learn about the oral method of instruction used by the Braidwoods in England failed because of their apparent reluctance to share such information, he visited the school founded by Abbé de l'Epée in France. Received cordially there by Abbé Sicard, successor to the founder, he learned the principles of the sign language that de l'Epée had introduced earlier. This was the method with which he returned to the United States to be used in the new Hartford school. The American School became the forerunner of the system of state-supported residential schools, providing the primary source of public education for deaf children in this country until well into the present century.

Meanwhile, a movement was spreading in New England requesting an alternative type of school confined exclusively to the oral method of instruction for those deaf children showing potential for oral communication. Influential proponents of this concept were able to establish the first permanent oral school in America, the Clarke School for the Deaf, which opened in 1867 in Northampton, MA. In the latter half of the 19th century, Alexander Graham Bell's efforts to promote the teaching of speech to the deaf also resulted in the founding of the Volta Bureau in Washington, DC to disseminate information about deafness and to promote the use of speech and residual hearing by the deaf. Bell's invention of the telephone in 1876, demonstrating the principles of electrical transmission of sound, paved the way for the development of the electronic hearing aid, representing perhaps the most significant "breakthrough" ever to occur for the hearing-impaired population.

With the population increasing and spreading westward, the number of hearing-impaired children also increased, and more educational facilities were required. Almost every state established its own public residential school to offer all deaf children residing within its boundaries an opportunity for an education. The manual method and, later, the combined method (oral and manual simultaneously) tended to evolve as the dominant method of instruction in public residential schools, while private residential schools were more often likely to offer an exclusively oral method of instruction.

By the beginning of this century a growing movement was underway to establish day programs for hearing-impaired children as an alternate setting. Many parents found the residential school objectionable because of the limitations imposed for integration of their children into daily family living. The first day programs were initiated in the larger city public school systems (Boston, New York, and Chicago). Here there were sufficient numbers of hearing-impaired children to make possible graded classes enabling satisfactory grouping with peers of comparable age. At first, such programs were conceptualized primarily as segregated schools, or classes, that differed from the residential school chiefly in that the children lived at home and returned there each night. Opportunities to associate with normally hearing children were not necessarily the rule, even in day classes situated in regular schools where such associations would have easily been possible. Nonetheless, the growth of these programs represented an important development in the attitudes that had so long separated the handicapped child from the rest of the public education system.

The rapid increase in the development of special education programs for hearing-impaired children in local education agencies across the nation has been quite remarkable when one considers that less than 25 years ago, Frisina (1959) reported twice as many such children being educated in residential schools (16,523) as in day programs (8,792). As a result of a national survey conducted in 1974-75, Rawlings and Trybus (1978) estimated that a total of 69,000 children were receiving special education services of

TABLE 8-1
Types of Educational Programs for Hearing-Impaired Children by Number and Enrollment, 1974-75

Program Type	Number of Programs	Total Enrollment	Total % of Enrollment
Residential schools for the deaf	69	19,521	32
Residential schools for the multiply handicapped	41	2,435	4
Day schools for the deaf	76	7,513	13
Day schools for the multiply handicapped	25	2,349	4
School districts offering full-time classes only	129	4,365	7
School districts offering part-time classes and services[a]	436	24,138	40
Total all programs	776	60,231	100%

Note: From F. H. Bess and F. E. McConnell, (1981). *Audiology, Education, and the Hearing Impaired Child*, C. V. Mosby, St. Louis, MO. Used with permission.

[a]Might also have included full-time classes.

some degree in schools across the nation during that school year. This estimate included almost 9,000 for whom no responses were forthcoming in their survey. Using the data from this survey, Bess and McConnell (1981) listed the distribution of enrollment by types of programs, showing that only 36% of more than 60,000 hearing-impaired children were being educated in residential schools in 1974-75 (Table 8-1). The growth of programs in local education agencies is evidence of the increased awareness of responsibility to the handicapped child on the part of educators and administrators, even though many of these programs may have been substantially lacking in appropriate standards.

Access to an Appropriate Education

The child who cannot hear, or who hears only partially, is at great disadvantage in the classroom. Imparting of information from teacher to pupil and from pupil to pupil relies primarily upon the use of the auditory modality. Although vision plays a vital role, it is secondary to hearing. One needs only to watch a television set with the sound tuned out to appreciate what many hearing-impaired children experience in the classroom. It then becomes apparent that communication through hearing, which is so natural and automatic that it is not given a passing thought by most teachers, is available only in part, or not at all, for the teacher of a hearing-impaired child. Truly, the educational barrier created by a hearing loss almost defies comprehension by those with normal hearing.

Establishment of Legal Precedents

In the preceding section, we have seen that from ancient times a separate set of rights with many legal restrictions developed for those whose severity of hearing impairment occurred at birth or early in life (thereby causing them to be classified as "deaf and dumb") as contrasted with those who were deafened in later life and thus retained their ability to speak ("deaf but not dumb"). The development of the concept that education could become a right did not occur until long after the earliest evidence that deaf children could be educated began to accumulate during and after the Renaissance period. In this country, the development of public residential schools and a smaller number of private schools in the 19th century, however, attested to a growing recognition that educational opportunity should be provided the child suffering severe hearing loss.

It was not until 1954 that education as a right received the legal sanction of the United States Supreme Court. Breunig and Nix (1977) cited the ruling handed down in the case of Brown v. Board of Education: "In these days, it is doubtful that any child may reasonably expect to succeed in life if he is denied the opportunity of an education. Such an opportunity, where the State has undertaken to provide it, is a right which must be made available to all on equal terms." Following this ruling, two decades of intensive effort by advocates of handicapped children occurred to win support in the Congress for the Education for All Handicapped Children Act of 1975 (PL 94-142) that was passed and signed into law on November 29, 1975. Its specifications regarding the rights and protections of handicapped children, including the hearing impaired, and their parents made it the most significant piece of legislation regarding the education of handicapped children ever to be passed. Breunig and Nix (1977) highlighted the need for such legislation by reporting congressional findings in 1975 to the effect that (1) more than half the handicapped children in the United States were not receiving appropriate educational services enabling them to have full equality of opportunity; and (2) as many as one million of the handicapped children in this country were being excluded entirely from the public school system.

The significance of the act for hearing-impaired children may be seen from a brief discussion of its major features and provisions, which are set forth in greater detail by Ballard and Zettel (1977) and by Bess and McConnell (1981). Among the major purposes of the act are (1) to guarantee the availability of a special education program to all handicapped children and youth who require it, without regard to such factors as region of geographic residence (which contributed to many inequities of opportunity in the past); (2) to assure fair and appropriate decision making relating to the provision of special education to handicapped children and youth; and (3) to assist the efforts of state and local government units through the use of federal funds. It defines handicapped children to include both the deaf and the hard-of-hearing, who by reason of their handicap require special education and related services. Special education is defined as specially designed instruction, at no cost to parents or guardians, to meet the unique needs of a handicapped child. Ballard and Zettel (1977) state the definition clearly implies that special education is derived "from the basic goals and expected outcomes of general education." Intervention for a hard-of-hearing child, for example, does not occur because the child is hard-of-hearing, but because the child has a unique educational need that requires specially designed instruction to help overcome the effects of the handicap in the educational setting.

The act further makes clear that handicapped children may require *related services*, even though some of these might not be available within the school system itself. Included here are diagnostic medical services, speech pathology and audiology, and psychological and counseling services. Such a provision has important implications, for example, in maintaining effective use of amplification for the hearing-impaired child, particularly in school systems lacking adequate audiologic personnel and services. Through contractual arrangements with an audiology clinic, ongoing audiologic management and inservice training of educational personnel can be obtained to ensure that the child derives the anticipated amount of functional hearing from the hearing aid. This, in turn, makes the instruction from the special teacher maximally effective.

In guaranteeing the right to a free appropriate public education, Public Law 94-142 stipulated an individualized education program (IEP) for each child. The IEP defines "appropriate" for each child, and it must be agreed upon by all parties (school and parents). It is crucial to the concept of

the act because it mandates that the education program must be addressed to the educational needs of a single child, rather than a class or group
of children. The importance of this provision for hearing-impaired children
is readily apparent, in view of the considerable number of factors that in
themselves present a wide range of variance in any group of children.
Although degree of hearing loss is a major such factor, highly interrelated
are those of age at onset, availability of early detection and intervention
programs in the infant years, use of hearing aids, family background, and
preschool training. Abeson and Winetraub (1977) point out that the IEP
is clearly intended as a "management device linking the child and appropriate services." Development of the IEP must precede placement in
a special education program, the specifics of which are delineated in the
IEP.

One additional element that merits mention is the provision in PL 94-142
that, to the maximum extent appropriate, handicapped children should
be educated with children who are not handicapped. Separation from the
regular educational environment is justifiable only when the nature or
severity of the individual handicap is such that education in regular classes
with supplementary services cannot meet the child's needs. This concept
has become known as the least restrictive alternative, and its interpretation obviously is subject to extremism from one end of the continuum to
the other; many of these interpretations may no doubt go far beyond the
act's intent.

A review of the provisions of PL 94-142 reveals, without question, that
the needs of hearing-impaired children have been addressed more specifically than ever before. Its passage marked the culmination of a decade of
progress in establishing the right to a free appropriate special education
and related services for all handicapped children. Although there remain
issues of policy that require more effective resolutions, a greater issue in
the 1980s is the very survival of this landmark federal legislation addressing itself specifically to the rights and protections of handicapped children
and their parents. Implementation of PL 94-142 was set for September 1,
1978, in order to give education systems a reasonable period of time to
prepare for some of its far-reaching provisions, many of which had not
been previously administered in the public schools. Within less than 3 years
of its implementation, however, the Education for All Handicapped
Children Act fell into danger of being repealed by the Department of
Education's proposed Elementary and Secondary Education Consolida-
tion Act of 1981. This legislation, emanating from the federal government's
objectives of paring government expenditures in order to help reduce in-
flation, grouped together 44 education programs into two block grants that
would give state and local governments considerable autonomy in how

federal funds would be used (Alexander Graham Bell Association for the Deaf, 1981). For example, money once targeted only for handicapped programs could be spent on any other educational program in the same "block." Thus, PL 94-142, representing 15 years of negotiations, discussion, and agreements worked out at the federal level to remedy special problems, was about to be repealed. Furthermore, no substitute was provided for even the right to an education. In fact, all rights, protections, and procedures, including child find and early identification, nondiscriminatory assessment, individualized education programs, education in the least restrictive environment, and procedures for resolving disputes of identification or placement decisions would have been eliminated (Ballard, 1981).

Fortunately, for hearing-impaired as well as other handicapped children, the Congress after careful consideration spared PL 94-142 from repeal by retaining it as a categorical program (and eliminating it from the block grant programs). This action was in response to an intense grassroots lobbying effort from individuals and organizations concerned with the handicapped across the United States. This experience indicates that constant vigilance and continued attempts to educate elected government officials will be required in the future to protect the gains that have already been made. The short time during which this legislation has been in effect, however, has already revealed certain shortcomings. Cumulative experience will reveal others. To serve the interests of hearing-impaired children, we need to amend and reform this important legislation, not rescind it altogether. In the words of an old saying, "Let us not throw out the baby with the bath water."

Role of Early Intervention

The question of whether legislation exists that would ensure opportunity for every hearing-impaired child to attain maximum language proficiency, full exploitation of residual hearing, and adequate communication skills requires that we look particularly at what has been done for the child in the years from birth to 6 years of age. More specifically, we now know that for those children with severe impairment, the 0-3 years period is critical. This position is no longer just a theoretical one; experience obtained in the past two decades in a number of programs for parents and infants in those prenursery school years has validated parent-infant intervention. Hayden (1979) points out that while nonhandicapped young children may make acceptable progress without early educational interventions, handicapped or at-risk children do not. To deny them the assistance that might increase their chances for improved functioning is, Hayden says, "not only wasteful," but "also ethically indefensible."

As for the hearing-impaired child, educators and audiologists appear to be well agreed that establishment of a language system in the first years of life, whether visual or auditory, is essential for the optimum cognitive functioning of the child throughout life. This view is supported by Lenneberg (1970), who postulates that the brain's function is best suited to learning language in the early period of life, and, in fact, that the brain itself is not quite mature as long as language is learned with ease. Because the normally hearing infant learns to make refined sound discriminations very early, Whetnall and Fry (1964) contended that the hearing-impaired child should have, from the first year of life, the opportunity to have his poor hearing boosted by use of a suitable hearing aid. They maintained that much of the severe handicap of deafness, insofar as speech and language are concerned, could be greatly ameliorated, even if not eliminated, if residual hearing were boosted with wearable hearing aids for all young deaf children in their first 18 months. Among the growing numbers of those whose experience and investigations support this view are Griffiths (1967), Pollack (1970), Northcott (1973), Castle and Warchol (1974), Calvert and Silverman (1975), Horton (1975), McConnell and Liff (1975), Beebe (1976), Ling (1976), Ross (1976), Fry (1977), and Bess and McConnell (1981).

Despite the well-documented significance of these first years of life in the hearing-impaired child's optimum cognitive and language development, the exclusion of children 0-3 years from the provisions of Public Law 94-142 has been noted with grave concern (Bess & McConnell, 1981; Hayden, 1979). Hayden, commenting that this exclusion raises some basic human issues as society strives for human rights, asks, "How old does a child have to be to have rights?" She concedes that the framers of the legislation may have been influenced in this decision not to include the infant handicapped population because of the anticipated complexity of developing a coordinated school-based program for this age group. Yet she fears the possibility that the decision reflected continuing resistance to the idea that such young children and their parents can indeed benefit from early educational intervention.

Furthermore, not only is a free appropriate public education for children 0-3 years unavailable in the provisions of the 1975 act, it also qualifies its mandate for children 3 through 5 years in these words:

Except that with respect to handicapped children aged 3 through 5 and aged 18 to 21, inclusive, the requirements of this clause shall not be applied in any State if the application of such requirements would be inconsistent with State law or practice, or the order of any court, respecting public education within such age groups in the State (Public Law [P. L.] 94-142, Section 612 [2] [B], 1975).

FIGURE 8-1
A hearing impaired child of 13 months learns to identify common household sounds in a parent/teaching home program

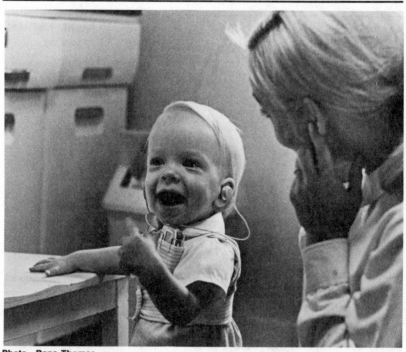

Photo—Dana Thomas

The foregoing exception could prevent the older handicapped preschoolers (age 3 through 5) in some states from receiving the educational opportunities critically needed. Fortunately, an amendment was added creating the Preschool Incentive Grant Program, *enabling*, but *not requiring*, states to request funding assistance to initiate, improve, and expand services to children in this age range (Cohen, Semmes, & Guralnick, 1979). Similarly, the Education Amendments of 1974, PL 93-380, gave support to education of children from birth through 21 years by requiring the states to set a goal for serving all handicapped children in this age range. No deadline, however, was given to delineate *when*, or *if*, the states must begin serving children aged 0-3 years.

The marked variability existing among the various states with respect to defining and identifying preschool handicapped children and determining their special education needs is made apparent from the results of a

TABLE 8-2
Variability Existing Among State Education Departments Regarding the Specification of an Age Criterion for Serving Preschool Handicapped Children

Age category	Number of states reporting
No age specified	17
3 years or above	11
Below school age or below 5 years	5
0-6 years	5
Variable by category	3
Deaf: 6 mo. All others—3-5 yr.	(1)
Hrng. impaired: 2.6 yr. All others—3-6 yr.	(1)
Deaf: 3 yr. All others—4 yr.	(1)
Under 21 yr.	2
4 years or older	1
Total states responding	44

Note: Data from Lessen and Rose, 1980.

survey conducted by Lessen and Rose (1980). They sought to determine from each of the 50 states (1) their definition, if any, of the preschool handicapped, and (2) their existing guidelines for the identification and placement of the preschool handicapped population. A questionnaire was mailed to the state consultants identified as being responsible for education of preschool handicapped children in each state. Responses were returned from 44 states. Less than one-third reported the inclusion of children down to birth (as designated by either "0-6," "below school age," "below 5," or "under 21"). The wide discrepancy from state to state is evidenced by the categorization of the 44 responses appearing in Table 8-2. Although no age is specified by 17 states, 13 others actually preclude children below 3 years, and in one other instance, below 2½ years.

When one considers the impact of this lack of emphasis in general on educational intervention for handicapped infants and nursery-age children, it is not surprising that the Council for Exceptional Children in its Bicentennial report to the White House Conference on Handicapped Individuals estimated that no more than 25% of preschool handicapped children nationwide were receiving "appropriate specialized educational services" (Hayden, 1979). Bess and McConnell (1981), in their analysis of data reported from the Annual Survey of Hearing Impaired Children and Youth, also emphasized that hearing-impaired children of school age are more likely than preschoolers to be enrolled in an educational intervention program of some sort. They cited data from Rawlings (1973), in which she reported on the age breakdown of 41,109 hearing impaired children enrolled in special education programs during the 1970-71 school year. Ninety-three percent of the children in this population were known to have been hearing impaired at birth or to have incurred their loss before age 3, and yet an extremely small proportion of these children receiving special education services were under 3. Further, children 6 through 13 years of age comprised more than five times the number of children 0-6 years who were receiving services.

The picture improves among the preschool population as age increases from three through five years, according to data from Murphy (1972). In a study of characteristics of preschool hearing-impaired children who were enrolled in special education programs, he found the number increased markedly each year as school age approached. From a total of 6,378 children in the survey, the proportions by age are shown in Table 8-3. It may be seen that more than half of all children in the survey were 5 years old, with the number in educational intervention placement steadily diminishing each year for children down to infancy. Commenting on the shortfall of educational intervention services for infant and nursery age hearing-impaired children, Bess and McConnell (1981) noted there is no evidence to cause us to conclude that the prevalence of hearing loss in young children is on the decline. Thus, the results of this survey substantiates that the numbers of children being detected and channeled into remedial programs at an early age (3 years and under) are not commensurate with the numbers of such children requiring such services. This situation confirms the point made earlier in this chapter that identification programs of hearing screening for newborns, infants, and preschoolers are neither consistent, uniform, nor easily available. There is a great need to overcome the apparent apathy that prevails in this area of health services for children.

Policy Issues Needing Reform

The accomplishment of a federal mandate to ensure that states and local school districts provide equal educational opportunities for handicapped children does not automatically achieve that goal at all levels of organization within the schools. And so it has already proven with the provisions of Public Law 94-142. Joiner and Sabatino (1981) point out that this act

TABLE 8-3
Distribution by Age of Hearing-impaired Children Under 6 Receiving Educational Services, United States: 1969-70.

Age (yrs.)	No. Children	Percent of Total
Under 3	336	5.2
3	699	11.0
4	1,865	29.3
5	3,478	54.5
Total	6,378	100.0

Note: Data from N. J. Murphy (1972). *Characteristics of hearing impaired students under six years of age, United States: 1969-70*, Series D, No. 7, Annual Survey of Hearing Impaired Children and Youth (Office of Demographic Studies, Gallaudet College, Washington, D.C.).

may be characterized as a "trickle-down" legislative and judicial intervention, with the government setting goals for school districts and maintaining control of funding once compliance is achieved. School administrators resistant to change can thwart the goal accomplishment through initiating change only in technical matters delineated by procedural details. Educators, they say, necessarily prioritize practices according to "levels of consciousness." It is significant that their study of professional educators' levels of consciousness for policies specified in PL 94-142 showed the lowest level was demonstrated by general education administrators. The majority of these administrators were building principals. As long as this kind of situation prevails, it is clear that setting the tone for acceptance of hearing-impaired children by general educators is in jeopardy. Thus, the general education administrators must become a principal target group for elevating consciousness levels by special educators to avoid the imminent polarization of special and general educators.

A second major area to which reform efforts need to be directed is that of the Individualized Education Program (IEP) conference participation. The IEP, a major component of the Education for All Handicapped Children Act, was designed to be a protection to handicapped children and their parents. Specifically, it mandates that the instruction program be addressed to the educational needs of a single child, rather than a class or group of children. No educational placement is to be undertaken until a written IEP has been drafted and agreed upon in the presence of those who have the most information about the child—that is, the parents and the teacher. Scanlon, Arick, and Phelps (1981) undertook a study in the Oregon schools to determine the nature and adequacy of IEP conference attendance and participation. They found a low attendance rate on the part of the regular classroom teacher and resource personnel and concluded that an open and supportive communication system between the regular and special educator, a necessary element of successful mainstreaming, was not being developed. The low attendance figures for all personnel other than the parent and the special educator implied that the implementation of the act was not in accord with the act's intent.

On the other hand, despite the good attendance participation by parents, they tend to have less influence on IEP decisions than warranted, according to Gilliam and Coleman (1981). They found a hierarchy of influence emerging that favored the participants who contributed more hard data, such as test scores, diagnostic reports, and cumulative records. To improve the IEP process in this regard, they recommend involving parents in the assessment and data-gathering phase. Parents are in a position to evaluate certain important areas of the child's functioning outside of school and to help identify specific needs for their child.

Perhaps the most perplexing issue in the implementation of the Education for All Handicapped Children Act has been the misconceptualizations surrounding the term "least restrictive environment." In essence, the act upholds the important principle that the integration of handicapped children and nonhandicapped children is, and should be, a much-desired goal of all special education. This principle is not new. As long as 20 years ago, Reynolds (1962) stated that preserving normal home and school life is a prevailing concept of special education, and that when special education is necessary, it should be no more "special" than necessary. He urged continuing assessment of children in special programs, so that they could be returned to more ordinary environments as early as possible. While there is an interlocking between least restrictive placement, normalization, and mainstreaming, they are not rigid mandates under PL 94-142; on the contrary, it, in fact, calls for flexibility and personalization in placement alternatives and opportunities (Dybwad, 1980). With respect to deaf children, Harrington (1974) pointed out that they must be considered quite differently from hard-of-hearing children in applying the mainstreaming process, the latter group being more likely to be suitable candidates for such placement if the appropriate supporting services are available. Lack of understanding on the part of overzealous advocates of mainstreaming can result in irreparable harm to hearing-impaired children who do not yet have the language proficiency and necessary communicative skills to compete with their hearing peers in a regular class.

Bess and McConnell (1981), in their discussion of this principle, conclude that the deciding factor for integrating hearing-impaired children into a regular classroom on either a part- or full-time basis rests on the facility with which they have mastered auditory-oral communication skills. If, for example, the child is primarily dependent upon manual communication skills, the inherent difficulties in exchanging information among the teacher, the hearing-impaired student, and his or her peers present significant barriers to the normal learning process. The nature of hearing impairment, and its effects on communicative functioning, can result in a completely isolated setting, both socially and emotionally, for many deaf and hard-of-hearing children if they are mainstreamed before they are ready. Proximity is not the same as integration.

In summary, the federally mandated law (PL 94-142) has been justifiably hailed as a great landmark in providing for the specialized needs of hearing-impaired children and helping them to realize the hopes and expectations they are capable of reaching. Yet, it is necessary for us to remember that the law is a continually changing and emerging process, and our challenge is not only to preserve the rights and protections this important legislation has guaranteed, but also to improve and extend its provisions through amendment and reform. A foremost consideration is to seek amendments to the act so that it includes children from birth to 3 years, and defines more stringently the provisions relating to children 3 through 5 years. Further, it has also been shown that a major effort to stem the threat of a growing breach between the general and special educator is needed. School administrators, in paritcular, should be included in orientation sessions designed to inform school personnel of the act's provisions and intent, and their more active participation invited and encouraged.

References

Abeson, A., & Winetraub, F. Understanding the individualized education program. In S. Torres (Ed.), *A primer on individualized education programs for handicapped children*. Reston, VA: Foundation for Exceptional Children, 1977.

Alexander Graham Bell Association for the Deaf. Congress saves P. L. 94-142 from block funding. *Newsounds*, 1981, *6*, 1; 5.

Ballard, J. (Ed.) Insight. The government report of the Council for Exceptional Children. *Update*, 1981, *12*, 5.

Ballard, J., & Zettel, J. Public Law 94-142 and Section 504: What they say about rights and protections, *Exceptional Children*, 1977, *44*, 177–185.

Beebe, H. H. Deaf children can learn to hear. In G. W. Nix (Ed.), *Mainstream education for hearing impaired children and youth*. New York: Grune & Stratton, 1976.

Bender, R. *The conquest of deafness*. Cleveland, OH: Press of Western Reserve University, 1960.

Bess, F. H., & McConnell, F. E. *Audiology, education and the hearing impaired child*. St. Louis: C. V. Mosby, 1981.

Breunig, H. L., & Nix, G. W. Historical and educational perspectives. *The Volta Review*, 1977, *79*, 263–269.

Calvert, D. R., & Silverman, S. R. *Speech and deafness* Washington, DC: Alexander Graham Bell Associaton for the Deaf, 1975.

Castle, D., & Warchol, B. Rochester's demonstration home program: A comprehensive parent infant program. *Peabody Journal of Education*, 1974, *51*, 73–80.

Cohen, S., Semmes, M., & Guralnick, M. J. Public Law 94-142 and the education of preschool handicapped children. *Exceptional Children*, 1979, *45*, 279–285.

Darley, F.L. (Ed.) Identification audiometry. *Journal of Speech and Hearing Disorders*, Monograph suppl. No. 9, 1961.

DeLand, F. *The story of lip-reading: Its genesis and development*. Washington, DC: The Volta Bureau, 1931.

Downs, M. Early identification of hearing loss: Where are we? Where do we go from here? In G. T. Mencher (Ed.), *Early identification of hearing loss*. Basel, Switzerland: A. G. Karger, 1976.

Downs, M. The expanding imperatives of early identification. In F. H. Bess (Ed.), *Childhood deafness: Causation, assessment, and management*. New York: Grune & Stratton, 1977.

Dybwad, G. Avoiding misconceptions of mainstreaming, the least restrictive environment, and normalization. *Exceptional Children*, 1980, *47*, 85–88.

Eagles, E. L., Wishik, S. M., Doerfler, L. G., Melnick, W., & Levine, H. S. *Hearing sensitivity and related factors in children*, St. Louis: Laryngoscope, 1963.

Frisina, D. R. Information concerning the deaf and hard of hearing in the United States. *American Annals of the Deaf*, 1959, *104*, 265–270.

Fry, D. B. Language development in the deaf child: A psycholinguist approach. In F. H. Bess (Ed.), *Childhood deafness: Causation, assessment, and management*. New York: Grune & Stratten, 1977.

Gilliam, J. E., & Coleman, M. C. Who influences IEP Committee decisions? *Exceptional Children*, 1981, *47*, 642–644.

Griffiths, C. *Conquering childhood deafness*, New York: Exposition Press, 1967.

Harrington, J. D. The integration of deaf children and youth through educational strategies. *Highlights* (Quarterly Bulletin, New York League for the Hard of Hearing), 1974, *53*, 6–8; 18.

Hayden, A. H. Handicapped children, birth to age 3. *Exceptional Children*, 1979, *45*, 510–516.

Horton, K. B. Early intervention through parent training. *Otolaryngologic Clinics of North America*, 1975, *8*, 143–157.

Horton, K. B. & Hanners, B. A. Trends in educational programming: The early years of the hearing impaired child, zero to three. In F. H. Bess (Ed.), *Childhood deafness: Causation, assessment, and management*. New York: Grune & Stratton, 1977.

Joiner, L. M., & Sabatino, D. A. A policy study of P. L. 94-142. *Exceptional Children*, 1981, *48*, 24–33.

Lenneberg, E. H. What is meant by a biological approach to language? *American Annals of the Deaf*, 1970, *115*, 67–72.

Lessen, E.I., & Rose, T.L. State definitions of preschool handicapped populations. *Exceptional Children*, 1980, *46*, 467–469.

Ling, D. *Speech and the hearing-impaired child*, Washington, DC: Alexander Graham Bell Association for the Deaf, 1976.

McConnell, F., & Liff, S. A home teaching program for parents of very young deaf children. *Otolaryngologic Clinics of North America*, 1975, *8*, 77–87.

Mencher, G.T. Screening the newborn infant for hearing loss: A complete identification program. In F.H. Bess (Ed.), *Childhood deafness: Causation, assessment, and management.* New York: Grune & Stratton, 1977.

Murphy, N.J. *Characteristics of hearing impaired students under six years of age, United States: 1969-70,* Series D, No. 7, Annual Survey of Hearing Impaired Children and Youth (Office of Demographic Studies, Gallaudet College, Washington, DC), 1972.

Northcott, W.H. Implementing programs for young hearing impaired children, *Exceptional Children,* 1973, *39,* 455-463.

Pollack, D. *Educational audiology for the limited hearing infant.* Springfield, IL: Charles C. Thomas, 1970.

Reynolds, M.C. A framework for considering some issues in special education, *Exceptional Children,* 1962, *28,* 367-370.

Rawlings, B. *Characteristics of hearing impaired students by hearing status. United States: 1970-71,* Series D, No. 10, Annual Survey of Hearing Impaired Children and Youth (Office of Demographic Studies, Gallaudet College, Washington, DC), 1973.

Rawlings, B.W., & Trybus, R.J. Personnel, facilities, and services available in schools and classes for hearing impaired children in the United States. *American Annals of the Deaf,* 1978, *123,* 99-114.

Ross, M. Model educational cascade for hearing impaired children. In G.W. Nix (Ed.), *Mainstream education for hearing impaired children and youth.* New York: Grune & Stratton, 1976.

Scanlon, C.A., Arick, J., & Phelps, N. Participation in the development of the IEP: Parents' perspective. *Exceptional Children,* 1981, *47,* 373-374.

Silverman, S.R. From Aristotle to Bell—and beyond. In H. Davis & S.R. Silverman (Eds.), *Hearing and deafness* (3rd ed.), New York: Holt, Rinehart & Winston, 1970.

Whetnall, E., & Fry, D.B. *The deaf child,* Springfield, IL: Charles C. Thomas, 1964.

Author Index

SUBJECT INDEX